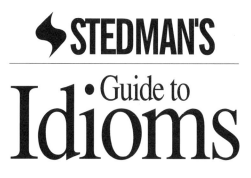

STEDMAN'S

Idioms •Guide to

KNOW THE LINGO

Elaine Olson, CMT, FAAMT

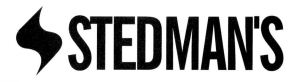

STEDMAN'S

Idioms •Guide to

KNOW THE LINGO

Elaine Olson, CMT, FAAMT

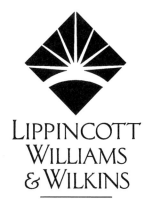

LIPPINCOTT
WILLIAMS
& WILKINS

Publisher: Julie K. Stegman
Managing Editor: Heather A. Rybacki
Production Coordinator: Jason Delaney
Associate Marketing Manager: Yvonne Palmer
Illustrator: Matt Andrews
Typesetter: Josephine Bergin
Printer & Binder: Malloy Litho, Inc.

Copyright © 2005 Lippincott Williams & Wilkins
351 West Camden Street
Baltimore, Maryland 21201-2436

Printed in the United States of America

First Edition, 2005

Library of Congress Cataloging-in-Publication Data

Olson, Elaine.Stedman's guide to idioms : know the lingo / Elaine Olson.
   p. ; cm.
Includes bibliographical references.
  ISBN 0-7817-5746-0
    1. Medicine—Terminology. 2. Medicine—Slang—Dictionaries.
3. English language—Idioms—Dictionaries. 4. Medical transcription—Terminology.
    [DNLM: 1. Medicine—Phrases—English. 2. Linguistics—Phrases—English. 3. Medical Records—Phrases—English. W 15 O52s 2005] I. Title: Guide to idioms. II. Title.

R123.O45 2005
610'.3—dc22

                                   2004028217
                                        01
                 1 2 3 4 5 6 7 8 9 10

Contents

Preface

America has long had a love relationship with words. Our language reflects our status as the melting pot of many cultures and backgrounds: We change the accent on a syllable of a foreign word, shorten a phrase, or take a formal saying or proverb and create a slang expression. This practice actually had its beginnings over a hundred years ago. People would quote a Bible passage or an adage, but give it a slightly different meaning than what was originally intended. For example, "What you sow, you reap," originally referred to being rewarded for one's efforts. But over the years, it came to mean, "What goes around comes around!"

Most of us in America grew up hearing our grandparents and parents using idioms, and now they are second nature to us. If you don't believe me, monitor your own conversations. You will be surprised how many idioms you use in just a few minutes.

In working with medical transcriptionists, I realized that even though they were learning the medical content of documentation, they were challenged with the idioms and slang phrases often scattered throughout the text. It became increasingly obvious that medical transcription not only encompasses anatomy and physiology, pharmaceuticals, surgical procedures, and various treatments, it also includes those everyday sayings that Americans are famous for: idioms. The challenge comes when the transcriptionist is not sure if what he or she heard was actually correct because the phrase does not fit the medical context of the document. This book is a result of many hours of developing workshops on idioms to help medical transcriptionists meet this challenge.

To demonstrate likely usages in medical dictation, the examples provided have been placed in that context when possible. When that was not feasible, a generic example was given.

And, even though this book is the outcome of working with medical transcriptionists, it is my hope that everyone who has been confounded by "one of those American sayings" will enjoy reading it, and it will find a place among your valued references.

Elaine Olson, CMT, FAAMT

Acknowledgments

What an incredible opportunity, to publish a book. It is a team effort with the collective talents of individuals who, for the most part, work in the background and do what they do best.

I would like to thank Lippincott Williams & Wilkins for this opportunity. Working with Publisher Julie K. Stegman, Managing Editor Heather A. Rybacki, and Production Coordinator Jason Delaney has been a wonderful experience for me.

A special thank you to Matt Andrews, Graphic Artist, who has provided humor through his graphic illustrations of some of the idioms. Matt, you are so talented and it has been a pleasure working with you.

Thank you Sandy Kovaks, CMT, FAAMT, for the final manuscript review. Sandy, your skills and sharp eye have kept me on the straight and narrow. Many thanks for being willing to work on this book with me.

My appreciation also goes to the following reviewers, who took the time to consider this book idea and provide their input: Catherine Anderson, AMRA; Debbie Askin, MN; Mary Bobik, CMT; Sharon Farley; Susan Francis, CMT, FAAMT; Ron Holliday, CMT; Lisa Nagle, BSed, CMA; Cindy Parman, CPC, CPC-H, RCC; Wendy Ryan, RHIT; Janet Stiles, BSN; Arlaine Walsh, CMT; and Julie Williams, CMT.

I would also like to thank some very special friends for their encouragement, support, and unwavering belief in me: Susan Francis, CMT, FAAMT; Bonnie Bakal, CMT, FAAMT; Pat Forbis, CMT, FAAMT; Carrie Donathan, CMT, FAAMT; Kathy Kropko, CMT, FAAMT; Julie Barnett, PT; and Jan Haney.

Elaine Olson, CMT, FAAMT

References

Merriam-Webster Online Dictionary. Available at www.m-w.com.

Spears, RA. *NTC's American Idioms Dictionary.* 3rd ed. Chicago, IL: NTC Publishing Group; 2000.

Dedicated to

Jason and Teri, I love you both very much

My mom, who gave me wings

Stella, the wind beneath my wings

and

in loving memory of

John Conrad Olson, DO,

who was blessed to be a blessing.

A

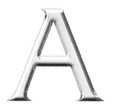

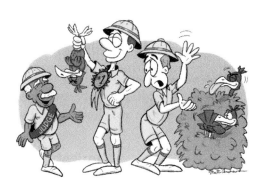

*A bird in the hand is
worth two in the bush*

Abide by (something)

To obey or comply.

Dr. Ming expects the patient to abide by his orders.

A bird in the hand is worth two in the bush

What you already have is better than what you might be
promised.

*Though proposed therapies might offer more suc-
cess, Ronnie decided to stay on the treatment already established. After all, a bird in the hand is
worth two in the bush.*

Able to breathe (easily or freely) again *or* Able to breathe a little easier

Able to relax or recover after a stressful situation.

The patient's life is no longer in danger; we are able to breathe a little easier now.

Able to take just so much

To have a limited amount of tolerance for something.

At the patient's request, we've increased her morphine dosage, as she is only able to take just so much pain.

Above and beyond

More than is required.

The EMS went above and beyond the call of duty to save the victim's life.

According to all accounts

From the reports given on a certain subject.

According to all accounts, the patient had been given optimal care during his hospital stay.

According to Hoyle

According to the rules; *Hoyle's Rules of Games* are considered the definitive set of rules governing card games.

The clinical trial was completed according to Hoyle in the hopes of receiving FDA approval for the drug.

Achilles' heel

A weakness that appears to be small but actually leads to one's downfall.

Mrs. Fraser always joked about how much she loved to eat candy, but her love of sweets turned into her Achilles' heel when she was diagnosed with diabetes.

Across the board

Equal for everyone.

Implementation of the electronic medical record will lead to improved health care across the board.

Act of faith

An act or deed demonstrating religious faith or a deep trust in someone or something.

It was an act of faith for the patient to have trusted the doctor.

Act of God

An occurrence for which no human is responsible.

If the patient recovers from his injuries, it will be an act of God.

Act up

To misbehave; to behave badly.

The patient acted up in the group counseling session and was immediately taken back to the ward.

Add fuel to the fire

To make a bad situation worse.

It only added fuel to the fire when the university locked down the campus after two students came down with meningococcal meningitis.

Add insult to injury

To make a bad situation worse.

To add insult to injury, the patient was then taken to the radiology department and unnecessarily x-rayed.

Advanced in years

Older in age.

Ms. Dewitt, who is advanced in years, has been admitted to the geriatric ward for observation.

After a fashion

In a manner that is just barely adequate; poorly.

The patient had been given treatment, after a fashion, with minimal results.

After all is said and done

When you consider everything that has been done; to summarize.

After all is said and done, the patient has done relatively well.

Against (someone's) will

Without permission or consent.

The patient was treated against her will.

Ahead of the game

To come out ahead of expectations.

This treatment puts us ahead of the game; we won't need to see the patient again for another two weeks.

Air (one's) dirty laundry

To share unpleasant secrets about yourself or others.

Beatrice seemed to enjoy airing her dirty laundry to whomever would listen.

Air (one's) grievances

To complain.

While completing her discharge forms, the patient began to air her grievances regarding the care she had received.

A little knowledge is a dangerous thing

Incomplete knowledge can cause damage or misunderstanding.

Patients often think they know enough to treat themselves, but a little knowledge is a dangerous thing when it comes to health care.

Alive and kicking

Healthy; animated.

Despite a long and difficult labor, the nurse was pleased to report to the waiting family that both the mother and the baby were alive and kicking.

Alive and well

Healthy; doing fine.

Dr. Johnson left the hospital several years ago to open a private practice, but he still stops by occasionally to let everyone know that he's alive and well.

All ears

Listening intently.

If you can come up with a better solution to the problem, then I'm all ears.

All for the best

Good despite the way it may seem.

The patient's condition quickly deteriorated, but it was all for the best. He would have never recovered fully from the extensive injuries.

All Greek to (someone)

Unintelligible; unable to understand.

Although the patient tried to listen carefully as his doctor explained the course of the illness, it was all Greek to him.

All hell broke loose

Everyone went crazy; chaos.

When the news anchor announced the hurricane was heading straight for the town, all hell broke loose as everyone tried to gather their things and leave.

All hours of the day

At any time of the day or night.

The emergency room is often swamped with patients all hours of the day.

All hours of the night

Very late into the night.

The colicky baby kept Maria up all hours of the night.

All joking aside *or* All kidding aside

To be serious for a moment.

All joking aside, the situation could have been quite serious.

All-out effort

A very thorough attempt.

An all-out effort was made to save the patient.

All skin and bones

Very thin.

The anorexic woman was all skin and bones.

All the same

Nevertheless; anyhow.

Miss Andrews appears to be fully recovered; all the same, the doctor will follow up with her in three weeks' time.

All thumbs

Clumsy.

I'm not sure why I signed up to take sewing lessons; when it comes to arts and crafts, I'm all thumbs.

All worked up

Excited or agitated about something.

The patient was all worked up over the change in the treatment plan.

An arm and a leg

A lot of money.

Physicians must pay an arm and a leg these days for insurance, thanks to the increase in malpractice lawsuits.

And the like

And other similar things.

The treatment plan consisted of medication, rest, proper diet, and the like.

Answer the call of nature

To use the bathroom.

The patient had to stop the therapy session to answer the call of nature.

Appear out of nowhere

To suddenly come into view.

According to the patient, the accident occurred

when a truck appeared out of nowhere and struck the side of her car.

Apples and oranges

Two entities that are not similar.

The patient's last admission and this admission are like apples and oranges; they simply cannot be compared.

Arrive on the scene

To appear in an area.

The ambulance was the last to arrive on the scene.

As a last resort

As the last choice.

Because of the many potential side effects, this new medication will be used only as a last resort.

As a matter of fact

Actually (in reference to what has just been said).

The patient stated that she is feeling well; as a matter of fact, she said she has not felt better in a long time.

As a rule *or* As a general rule

Usually; almost always.

As a rule, pregnant women are advised not to drink alcoholic beverages.

As bad as all that

As bad as reported; as bad as it seems.

Even though the patient was concerned about the test results, the doctor did not feel it was as bad as all that.

As big as life

An exaggerated way of saying a person or thing appeared in a particular place.

The patient appeared in my office, as big as life, and insisted on seeing me!

As blind as a bat

To have poor eyesight.

The elderly gentleman was as blind as a bat!

As clear as mud

Not understandable; unclear.

The patient's explanation was as clear as mud.

As different as night and day

Completely different.

Although the patient thought he had the same symptoms as last time, they were actually as different as night and day.

As far as anyone knows

To the limits of anyone's knowledge.

As far as anyone knows, this is the first time this patient has had this problem.

As flat as a pancake

Very flat.

The patient hurt his wrist when he smashed the bug as flat as a pancake.

As high as a kite

Extremely intoxicated.

While the patient claimed to be drug-free, it was obvious that he was as high as a kite during his counseling session.

As old as the hills *or* As old as dirt

Very old.

The practice of medicine is as old as the hills.

As plain as the nose on your face

Apparent; clear; not hidden or mysterious.

It should be as plain as the nose on your face that Maribeth isn't really ill; she is just pretending to be sick to get attention.

As quiet as a mouse

Very quiet.

Roger was as quiet as a mouse throughout the exam.

As regular as clockwork

Dependably regular.

Ms. Lopez said that her migraines occur as regular as clockwork.

As slippery as an eel

Devious; undependable.

The patient left the hospital unobserved. He is as slippery as an eel.

As stubborn as a mule

Very stubborn.

Mr. McCoy is as stubborn as a mule; he refuses to take his medication.

As white as a sheet

Very pale.

The patient arrived in the emergency department as white as a sheet.

Assault and battery

A violent attack.

The woman admitted this morning was the victim of an assault and battery.

At a loss (for words)

Unable to verbally respond to a statement or explain a situation.

The doctor was at a loss for words to explain the patient's miraculous recovery.

At all times

Constantly.

The patient is to be on oxygen at all times.

At any rate

Anyway.

At any rate, the patient is doing better, so we will continue as planned.

At death's door

Very close to dying or about to die.

Mr. Bertone was at death's door when his condition suddenly improved.

At heart

Deep down; one's true essence.

Dr. Antonetti can seem somewhat brusque when you first meet him, but he is truly a caring man at heart.

At once

Immediately.

Take the patient to the operating room at once.

At the end of (one's) rope

Frazzled or frustrated.

Marcus was at the end of his rope after standing in line for three hours only to be told that he was not eligible to receive the vaccination.

At the present time

Currently; now.

At the present time, all of the hospital beds are full.

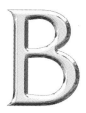

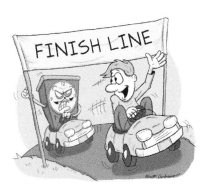

Beat the clock

Back East

To or from the eastern United States.

Upon discharge, the patient will be heading back East and will follow up with his regular physician.

Back-handed compliment

An insult disguised as a compliment.

Howard pays his wife a lot of backhanded compliments, but he does it in such a good-natured way that she doesn't take too much offense.

Back-to-back

Adjacent; touching.

The doctor has been so busy with this year's flu outbreak that he is seeing patients back-to-back all day without a break.

Be a must

A necessity; something that has to be done.

It is a must to have the patient return for followup.

Bear with (someone or something)

To be patient with someone or something.

Please bear with me while I fill out this form.

Beat around the bush

To avoid answering a question.

The patient kept beating around the bush to avoid discussing the actual problem.

Beat the clock

To do something before a deadline.

Ed arrived early to beat the clock.

Beef up (something)

To enhance; to make stronger.

We will try to beef up the treatment process to meet the patient's needs.

Been through the mill

Been treated badly.

After surgery, the patient looked like she had been through the mill.

Beg, borrow, or steal

To attain something through whatever means are necessary.

Antonio was prepared to beg, borrow, or steal to get in on the new clinical trial.

Beg off

To ask to be released from something.

The patient begged off from her PT appointment but will reschedule next week.

Behind the eight ball

In a difficult position.

Dr. Nikola hated to admit it, but he was really behind the eight ball trying to figure out the best course of action for Raphael.

Bend over backwards

To go out of one's way, often to accommodate someone else or to put someone else at ease.

The entire hospital staff bent over backwards to make a good impression when the nationally renowned surgeon visited.

Beside the point

Irrelevant.

The patient had other complaints, but they were beside the point.

Beyond a reasonable doubt

Almost without any doubt.

Treatment will continue until we have gone beyond a reasonable doubt that all efforts were made on the patient's behalf.

Bide (one's) time

To wait patiently.

Her condition is progressing as well as can be expected, but we will have to bide our time and see what the final outcome will be.

Blind leading the blind

A situation where someone who does not know something tries to explain it to someone else.

The patient's wife tried to explain the procedure to her husband, but it was like the blind leading the blind.

Blow over

To go away.

If we wait, the situation may blow over.

Boil down to (something)

To summarize.

What it boils down to is that the patient needs to go into surgery immediately.

Breathe easy

To assume a relaxed state after a stressful period.

We all breathed easy knowing Dr. Dimanti was in charge.

Bright and early

Very early.

The patient will be discharged bright and early tomorrow morning.

Bring home the bacon

To earn a salary.

The patient was concerned about the lengthy hospital stay since she is responsible for bringing home the bacon.

Buckle down

To approach a task with a new level of determination and focus.

We really need to buckle down and study if we hope to pass this test.

Bug (someone)

To irritate or bother someone.

If you're unsure of the answer, try looking it up in your references before you bug your co-workers about it.

Build a fire under (someone)

To motivate someone to do something.

I will have to build a fire under that nurse to get her to move faster!

Bundle of nerves

Someone who is very nervous.

The patient is a bundle of nerves over the impending surgery.

Burn (one's) bridges

To alienate one's relationships.

Al needs to learn not to burn his bridges, or he'll quickly find out how lonely he can be.

Burst into tears

To suddenly start to cry.

Elizabeth burst into tears when she heard the diagnosis.

Burst out laughing

To suddenly start to laugh.

The patient bordered on hysteria and burst out laughing several times during the interview.

Bury the hatchet

To let past disagreements go.

What do you say we bury the hatchet and try to be friends again?

By and large

Generally speaking.

By and large, the patient does what he is told to do.

By leaps and bounds

Rapidly; by large progressive steps.

The infant's condition improved by leaps and bounds in just a few days.

By the book

According to the accepted rules or guidelines.

The pharmaceutical company was anxious to get approval for the new cholesterol-lowering medication; however, they knew they had to do everything by the book to be considered by the FDA.

By the numbers

In a systematic or routine manner.

It took Dr. Hill over eight hours to complete the complicated procedure, but he wanted to make sure he took his time and did it by the numbers.

By the same token

In the same way.

Mr. Walters seems to be much more upbeat today, and by the same token, his wife appears to be in better spirits as well.

By the seat of (one's) pants

By sheer luck.

The patient made it to the hospital by the seat of his pants.

By the skin of (one's) teeth

By a narrow margin.

Marinda went into early labor but managed to make it to the hospital by the skin of her teeth.

By the sweat of (one's) brow

Through one's own hard work.

Adilene made it through medical school by the sweat of her brow.

By the way *or* By the by

To bring up a different topic.

By the way, if you see Mr. Munro, could you tell him I'm looking for him?

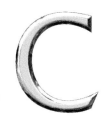

C

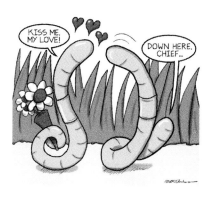

*Can't make heads
or tails of it*

Call a spade a spade

To speak frankly about something.

When discussing a patient's prognosis, Dr. Clark is always upfront, calling a spade a spade.

Call it a day

To quit what one is doing for the day.

After making rounds, the doctor is going to call it a day and go home.

Call it a night

To quit what one is doing at night and go home.

The EMS technicians had a particularly demanding shift and were ready to call it a night.

Call it quits

To discontinue something; give up.

Miguel did not want to pursue other courses of treatment, so he called it quits.

Call of nature

The need to use the restroom.

Miss O'Brien asked that we take a break from the therapy session so she could answer the call of nature.

Call (someone) down

To reprimand or scold.

The doctor had to call the patient down after he continued to drink while taking his medication.

Call (someone) on the carpet

To reprimand or scold.

The new resident was called on the carpet for habitually arriving late for rounds.

Call (someone or something) into question

To challenge the effectiveness or accuracy of something.

Based on reports of extensive side effects, the new protocol was called into question.

Call (someone or something) off

To stop an action from taking place or continuing.

The surgical rounds were called off due to an emergency.

Call (someone's) bluff

To demand that someone prove they can do what they say they can do.

Jake called Mark's bluff and insisted that he eat the whole pie.

Call (something) up

To bring information up on a computer system.

With the new integrated system, doctors can call up their patients' lab results from any computer in the hospital.

Call the shots

To make the decisions.

The surgeon will be calling the shots now that the patient is under her care.

Can't help but (do something)

Forced or compelled to do something or act in a certain way because of the surrounding circumstances.

You can't help but laugh when Dr. Millner starts telling stories about the antics he pulled in med school.

Can't hold a candle to (someone or something)

Not equal to someone or something; usually implies that the subject is superior to everything or everyone else in some respect.

No one can hold a candle to Bonnie; she is an expert in her field.

Can't make heads or tails of (someone or something)

Unable to figure someone or something out; stumped.

The referring physician was unable to make heads or tails of the chart; he had never seen a more disorganized document.

Can't see beyond the end of (one's) nose

Shortsighted; unable to see the bigger picture.

John has no idea what he is getting into; he can't see beyond the end of his nose!

Cards are stacked against (someone)

To have the odds again you; to be in a less than advantageous position.

When Martina was diagnosed with multiple sclerosis in addition to her existing cancer, she felt like the cards were stacked against her.

Carried away

Excited.

Dr. Francis tends to get a little carried away when discussing his research; he can go on about it for hours.

Carry a lot of weight

To be very influential.

Since he is chief of the cardiology department, Dr. Andrews' opinion carries a lot of weight.

Carry a torch for (someone)

To continue loving someone when they do not return the feeling.

Will is still carrying a torch for his ex-girlfriend.

Carry on about (something)

To make a great fuss over.

Like all new grandmothers, Jan loves to carry on about her granddaughter.

Carry on without (someone or something)

To manage to continue without someone or something.

Although she admits it has been difficult at times, Ms. Larew has managed to carry on after the death of her husband.

Carry (one's) own weight

To do one's share.

Everyone must carry his or her own weight for the project to succeed.

Carry out (something)

To perform a task.

We will carry out the testing next week when the patient is stronger.

Carry over (something)

To extend into another time period or location.

Angela's insurance coverage should carry over into next year.

Carry the weight of the world on (one's) shoulders

To appear to be burdened by all the problems in the world.

Nicolas tends to carry the weight of the world on his shoulders, which is certainly a contributing factor to his recent depression.

Carte blanche to (do something)

The freedom to do as one chooses.

The cardiologist was given carte blanche to treat the patient aggressively.

Case in point

For example.

The hospital changed protocol because of the many complaints it received, case in point, Mrs. Smith's rash.

Cast doubt on (something)

To cause someone or something to be distrusted.

Because the patient misled the staff about her symptoms, it cast doubt on her credibility.

Catch a cold (or other illness)

To contract a disease.

You sound like you have a bit of a cough. Are you catching a cold?

Catch fire

To ignite and burn.

Be careful when burning candles or your house could catch fire.

Catch forty winks

To get some sleep.

The resident wanted to catch forty winks before starting her next shift.

Catch it

To get in trouble.

If the patient is not compliant with his therapy, he will catch it from the doctor.

Catch on

To become readily accepted; usually refers to a fad, an idea, or a way of thinking.

Although it took awhile to catch on, it is now the norm to have fathers present in the delivery room.

Catch on (to something)

To figure something out.

While I know it can take awhile to get used to using crutches, I'm sure you'll catch on in no time.

Catch (one's) breath

To resume normal breathing pattern.

After the Bruce protocol, it took a little while for the patient to catch his breath.

Catch (someone) off guard

To surprise someone.

The test results caught the patient off guard, but he was very pleased.

Catch (someone) red-handed

To catch a person in the act of doing something wrong.

The dietician caught the patient red-handed. Despite strict orders to avoid sugary foods, she saw him at Krispy Kreme, gorging himself on donuts!

Cat got your tongue?

Are you unable to speak? (used jokingly)

Why won't you answer me? Has the cat got your tongue?

Caught in the cross fire

Caught between two arguing people or groups.

Dr. Jones did not want to be caught in the cross fire between the patient's wishes and her family's.

Caught in the middle of (something)

Caught between two arguing people or groups.

Although he would have preferred to be left out of

it, somehow Bill got caught in the middle of a debate about physician-assisted suicide.

Cause a commotion

To cause trouble; to start a disturbance.

It caused quite a commotion when the little girl's pet gerbil got loose in the ER.

Cause tongues to wag

To cause people to gossip.

Her outrageous behavior at the party caused tongues to wag!

Cease and desist

To permanently stop doing something; often suggests legal implications.

The court order required the hospital to cease and desist hiring illegal aliens.

Chalk (something) up to (something else)

To attribute a result to an action.

When the antibiotic failed to cure the infection, we chalked it up to a resistant strain of the virus and pursued other courses of treatment.

Change hands

For something to be passed from one person to another.

The care of the patient will change hands as soon as he is transferred.

Change (one's) tune

To change one's story or behavior, usually from untruthful to truthful, bad to good, or rude to pleasant.

When the drug test results came back positive, Missy changed her tune and admitted to occasional recreational drug use.

Chapter and verse

Detailed information on a particular subject.

The article on nerve damage gave chapter and verse for all possible treatments.

Charged up

Agitated; excited.

The patient got all charged up when he found out they were postponing his surgery once again.

Cheat on (someone or something)

To betray or be disloyal.

Nurse Martin scolded the patient after discovering that she had cheated on her diet.

Check in

To see to the welfare of someone or something.

I will check in on you later to see how you are doing.

Chew out (someone)

To scold someone.

The doctor chewed out the nurse for not notifying him earlier of the change in the patient's condition.

Child's play

Very easy; simple.

After dealing with such a difficult flu strain last winter, this year's flu season should be child's play.

Chilled to the bone

Very cold; can also imply extreme fright.

The patient was chilled to the bone, so the nurse gave her a heated blanket.

Choke up

On the verge of tears; to become emotional and speechless.

Ms. Campos always gets a little choked up when talking about the quality of care hospice provided for her husband.

Clam up

To shut up; stop talking.

The moment the police walked into the room, the gunshot victim clammed up.

Clean bill of health

In good physical condition.

After a complete physical exam, the doctor gave Courtney a clean bill of health.

Clean up (one's) act

To reform one's conduct.

The orderly was told to clean up his act if he wanted to keep his job.

Clear sailing

Progress made without any difficulty.

After the initial crisis, it was clear sailing, and the patient continued to make steady improvement.

Clear the air

To get rid of doubts or hard feelings.

Therapy sessions can be a good way to clear the air between a patient and their family.

Climb on the bandwagon

To join others in supporting someone or something.

Marcel felt confident that the new drug was effective and climbed on the bandwagon to promote it.

Clip (someone's) wings

To hold someone back; to take away one's freedom or privileges.

The doctor warned the resident that he would clip his wings if his patient care didn't improve.

Cloak-and-dagger

Involving secrecy.

The whole affair was cloak-and-dagger, and no one really knew what was going on.

Close at hand

Within reach.

The patient kept her heart medication close at hand.

Clue (someone) in

To inform someone of something.

Dr. Reyna clued Dr. Nils in on the patient's history of hypochondria.

Coast to coast

Across the United States; from the Atlantic Ocean to the Pacific Ocean.

The breakthrough cancer research made headlines from coast to coast.

Cold turkey

Abruptly stopping use of an addictive substance.

After 20 years of smoking, Marissa decided to go cold turkey and quit once and for all.

Come and gone

To arrive and leave; to have already passed.

The due date came and went, yet the hospital did nothing to ensure HIPAA compliance.

Come apart at the seams

To suddenly lose one's emotional control.

After the death of his mother, Bill came apart at the seams.

Come around

To finally agree.

After some persuasion, Mr. Huan came around to the doctor's way of thinking.

Come clean

To be honest.

The patient finally came clean about her involvement with drugs.

Come full circle

To return to the original position or state of affairs.

After many attempts at the new protocol, the patient had come full circle.

Come out of nowhere

To appear suddenly.

The patient's agitation seemed to come out of nowhere and can probably be attributed to a sudden drop in her blood sugar.

Come through with flying colors

To get through a situation extremely well.

Jim came through surgery with flying colors.

Come to a head

To reach a crucial point.

The situation has come to a head and must be addressed.

Come to an end

To stop; to finish.

The patient has reached maximum medical benefit, indicating that treatment has come to an end.

Come to blows

To fight about something.

There's no need to come to blows over a simple difference of opinion.

Come to mind

To remember something.

The hospital administrator asked Luann to call him if any other potential job candidates came to mind.

Conk out

To pass out; to go to sleep.

Joey was so tired after his PT session, he just conked out!

Cool your heels

Be patient; relax.

I will be there soon, so just cool your heels.

Cough up (something)

To produce something, usually money or the truth.

Mary had to cough up $80 to pay for her bill.

Couldn't care less

To not care at all.

Catherine was so depressed that she couldn't have cared less about her job or her family.

Cover a lot of ground

To travel a great distance; to investigate a wide range of information.

A lot of ground has been covered in researching the origin of the SARS virus.

Crack a book

To open a book to study.

Even though John never seems to crack a book, he's still a straight-A student.

Cream of the crop

The best there is.

In an effort to attract the cream of the crop, the hospital recruited graduates from the top medical schools across the country.

Cross that bridge when (one) comes to it

To deal with a problem only when one is face-to-face with it.

The patient is in denial about the severity of her condition and will need further therapy, but we will cross that bridge when we come to it.

Cruising for a bruising

Asking for trouble or a fight.

Even though she had had several warnings from the doctor to get plenty of rest, Brenda continued to overextend herself. She was really cruising for a bruising.

Crux of the matter

The central issue.

When Mr. Taylor was admitted with severe abdominal pain, Dr. Collins immediately went to work to discover the crux of the matter.

Cry wolf

To complain about something or make a big fuss when nothing is really wrong; to raise a false alarm.

Don't cry wolf if you want people to believe what you say.

Cue (someone) in

To prompt someone to do their part in a process.

After the patient was prepped and draped, the nurse cued the doctor in to begin surgery.

Cut and dry

Straightforward.

The appendectomy was cut and dry; there were no complications, and the patient was discharged within 48 hours.

Cut both ways

To affect both sides of the issue equally.

Implementing HIPAA regulations will cut both ways: patient privacy will be improved, but the increase in paperwork will lead to higher healthcare costs.

Cut corners

To take a shortcut; to do things poorly.

Cutting corners to save money may adversely affect patient care.

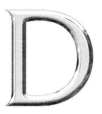

D

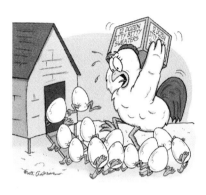

*Don't count your chickens
before they hatch*

Dance to another tune

To change an attitude, opinion, or behavior pattern.

After learning the truth, Martha danced to another tune.

Dare (someone) to do (something)

To challenge someone to do something that will test their courage or fortitude.

I dare you to climb that water tower.

Dark horse

Someone that has talents or plans that are not widely known.

Surprisingly, Emma ended up being the dark horse on the marketing team; she came up with an amazing plan for promoting the new equipment.

Dart in and out

To move quickly between two things.

The red car kept darting in and out of traffic.

Dash cold water on (something or someone)

To splash cold water on something or someone.

When Ms. Moore felt faint, her daughter dashed cold water on her face.

Date back

To extend back to a particular time.

The patient's back problems date back to a car accident she was involved in approximately five years ago.

Davy Jones's locker

The bottom of the sea.

The jewels and gold coins from the ship ended up in Davy Jones's locker.

Dawn on (someone)

To occur to someone.

It finally dawned on Susan that she would have to be compliant if she wanted to get better.

Day after day

Every day; all the time.

Mrs. Briscoe visits her husband at the nursing home day after day.

Dead duck

Someone or something in a hopeless situation.

If Jeff misses his flight again, he is a dead duck!

Devil-may-care attitude

Very casual attitude; carefree.

The patient had a devil-may-care attitude toward his prognosis and didn't take his treatment seriously.

Dime a dozen

Abundant; cheap; common.

Those pens are a dime a dozen.

Do a double take

To react with surprise; to look twice at something to be certain about what you saw.

The expectant mother did a double take when she saw triplets on the sonogram.

Do the trick

To do exactly what needs to be done.

The patient is still experiencing some discomfort, but the newly prescribed medication should do the trick.

Don't count your chickens before they hatch

Don't plan to use something before you actually have it.

Stephanie wants to go shopping before she gets her Christmas bonus, but she shouldn't count her chickens before they hatch!

Dose of (one's) own medicine

The same kind of treatment that one gives to other people.

Sally is overly critical of others; one of these days, someone will give her a dose of her own medicine.

Double up

To share something with someone.

There aren't enough books to go around, so some of the students will have to double up.

Down in the dumps

Sad or depressed.

After learning that she would not be released today, the patient was really down in the dumps.

Drop in the bucket

A very small amount, especially when compared to the overall picture.

The cost of cosmetic surgery was just a drop in the bucket to the wealthy movie producer.

Drop in the ocean

A very small amount, especially when compared to the overall picture.

Unfortunately, it appears that Miss Sawyer's persistent headaches are just a drop in the ocean when put in context with her other health problems.

Drop the ball

To make a mistake, usually because of lack of attention or focus.

It is crucial that no one drops the ball when caring for patients in the ICU.

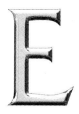

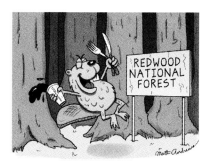

Eager beaver

Eager beaver

Someone who is very enthusiastic.

On his first day of residency, Paul seemed like an eager beaver, ready to pitch in wherever he was needed.

Eagle eye

Careful attention; an intently watchful eye.

The doctor kept an eagle eye on the patient's condition to watch for any subtle changes.

Early bird

Someone who habitually gets up early in the morning or arrives early.

Jonathan is such an early bird. He usually gets to the gym by 6 a.m.

Early on

In the beginning stages.

Because the doctor caught Marie's cancer early on, treatment should be effective.

Early to bed, early to rise, makes one healthy, wealthy, and wise.

A proverb that claims that going to bed early and getting up early is good for you; often shortened to "early to bed, early to rise."

Dr. Williams always recommends a good night's sleep to his patients, reminding them that early to bed, early to rise, makes one healthy, wealthy, and wise.

Ease off

To reduce the urgency or frequency with which one does something.

When Molly decided she wanted to ease off her antidepressant medication, her psychiatrist helped her taper down her dose safely.

Easier said than done

A task is simpler to talk about than it is to actually complete.

Given the patient's locale, emergency treatment was easier said than done.

Easy as apple pie

Not difficult at all.

Stella was afraid to go snowboarding, but soon found the beginner slopes easy as apple pie.

Easy as pie

Not difficult at all.

At first, Betty feared giving herself insulin injections, but soon she found it to be easy as pie.

Easy come, easy go

To lose something that took little effort to obtain in the first place.

The nutritionist told Becky that weight loss achieved from fad dieting is often easy come, easy go, and that healthy eating and exercise habits produce more lasting results.

Easy to come by

Readily available.

Data on the new drug was easy to come by on the Internet.

Eat and run

To consume a meal or a snack and then leave shortly afterwards.

Shane was late for his shift, so he had to eat and run.

Eat away at (someone or something)

To wear down, erode, or bother.

At her therapist's advice, Sue confronted Paul about her anger before it could eat away at her.

Eat high on the hog

To consume extravagant or expensive food.

The patient's cholesterol levels were elevated, a sure sign that he had been eating high on the hog.

Eat humble pie

To acknowledge that one has been proven wrong.

Barry didn't think the doctor's suggestion to meditate would help his stress levels, but after trying it, he felt better and had to eat humble pie.

Eat (one's) cake and have it too

To be able to take advantage of two seemingly contradictory things.

People often want to be healthier without giving up their bad habits, but you can't eat your cake and have it too.

Eat (one's) words

To retract one's statement.

Gary was positive he was right, but when Virginia proved otherwise, he had to eat his words.

Eat out of (someone's) hand

To obey or cooperate with someone.

The nurse's kind and gentle demeanor led patients to eat out of her hand and comply with whatever she asked of them.

Ebb and flow

To decrease and then increase.

The patient reported that his symptoms ebb and flow without warning.

Edge (someone) out

To competitively remove a person from a job, office, or position.

Joanne edged out Mark for the chief-of-staff position.

Egg (someone) on

To urge or dare someone to do something that is usually unwise.

Martin did not want to steal the car, but his friends egged him on until he did.

Either feast or famine

Either too much or too little.

The workload in medical transcription tends to be either feast or famine.

Eleventh hour

The last possible moment.

At the eleventh hour, when nothing else worked, Dr. Howard decided to operate on the patient.

End of the road

The final option or outcome of a situation.

There are simply no other treatment options, so it looks like this last round of chemotherapy is the end of the road for the patient.

End up (doing something)

To do something different than originally planned.

The initial treatment did not work, so the doctor ended up performing an invasive procedure.

End up with the short end of the stick

To have less than or to be in a worse situation than someone else.

Tom ended up with the short end of the stick when Larry took credit for his new idea.

Engage in small talk

To chat about minor matters.

The psychiatrist engaged the patient in small talk in an attempt to make her feel more comfortable.

Enough is enough

It is time to stop.

Ken's doctor told him that enough was enough when it came to eating so much fast food.

Enough to wake the dead

Extremely loud.

When the nurse knocked over the tray of surgical tools, the noise was enough to wake the dead.

Escape (someone's) notice

To go undetected.

My earlier memo must have escaped your notice, so I am sending you another one as a reminder.

Even in the best of times

When things are going well.

Even in the best of times it is difficult to find adequate nursing staff.

Every dog has his day

Everyone will get a chance to achieve success.

Your opportunity will come; after all, every dog has his day.

Every inch a (something)

Completely.

Roger is every inch a gentleman.

Every last one

The complete group or collection of something.

Dr. Coburn checked on every last one of his patients before he left for the night.

Every minute counts

Time is very important.

The patient's condition is so critical that every minute counts, so he must be taken to surgery immediately.

Every now and then

Occasionally; infrequently.

Every now and then the patient notices swelling in the right leg.

Every Tom, Dick, and Harry

Everyone inclusively, without discrimination.

The nursing supervisor was very strict and did not want every Tom, Dick, and Harry in the delivery suite.

Every which way

In all directions.

The patient complained that his abdominal pain went every which way.

Everything but the kitchen sink

Almost everything one can think of.

Susan is always prepared; she must have everything but the kitchen sink in her purse.

Explain (oneself)

To justify one's words, actions, or thoughts.

The doctor listened as the patient explained himself.

Extend sympathy

To express compassion.

Having told the patient of her prognosis, the doctor extended his sympathy to her family.

Extenuating circumstances

Special conditions.

Since the patient sustained the injury on hospital grounds, he was admitted under extenuating circumstances.

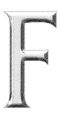

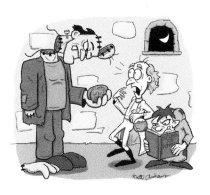

*Falling apart at the
seams*

Face (someone) down

To overcome someone by being bold.

When the patient suddenly became abusive, the doctor faced him down and took control of the situation.

Face the music

To accept the unpleasant results of one's own actions.

The patient didn't take all her medication and had to face the music when she relapsed.

Fair game

Someone or something that it is permissible to criticize or attack.

Politicians and movie stars know that the press considers them fair game.

Fair to middling

Average; acceptable.

The quality of the work was fair to middling.

Fair-weather friend

Someone who is only helpful or agreeable when things are going well.

Helen realized what a fair-weather friend Janine was when her car broke down and Janine refused to drive her to her doctor's appointment.

Fall apart at the seams

To lose control emotionally.

During his residency, Ruben was under such stress that he felt like he would fall apart at the seams.

Fall back on (someone or something)

To turn to someone or something for help as a last resort.

Dan preferred not to take antibiotics, but he got the prescription filled anyway, just in case he needed to fall back on them.

Fall by the wayside

To get lost amid all that is happening.

During the holiday season, it takes a lot of strength and determination to keep one's diet from falling by the wayside.

Fall down on the job

To fail to do something properly.

Nurses need intense medical training so that they don't fall down on the job.

Fall flat on (one's) face

To be completely unsuccessful.

If you do not prepare properly for your presentation, you might fall flat on your face!

Fall from grace

To cease to be held in favor, especially because of some wrong or foolish action.

The usually exemplary student fell from grace when he cheated on the exam.

Fall into a trap

To mistakenly trust someone or something.

The patient fell into the trap of believing that herbs would cure him rather than his prescribed medication.

Fall through

To not happen.

Unfortunately, the grant money fell through, so the researchers could not complete the study.

Falling out

An argument.

Marge and her brother had a falling out over her choice of rehab.

Familiarity breeds contempt

Knowing a person, process, or thing too well can lead to bad feelings.

Although he liked his workout routine at first, Ben found that, after several months, familiarity bred contempt, so he tried a combination of weight lifting, running, and aerobics.

Far and away

Unquestionably.

Dr. Rohan determined that a statin drug was far and away the best option to treat the patient's high cholesterol levels.

Far be it from (someone)

Inappropriate for someone to do or say something.

Far be it from me to tell the doctor what to prescribe for the patient.

Far cry from (something)

Very different from something else.

The treatment at the acute care facility was a far

cry from what the patient received at the rural clinic.

Fast and furious

Very rapid and with unrestrained energy.

Things move fast and furious in the emergency room when a trauma case arrives.

Fat chance

Very little likelihood.

Fat chance that this difficult patient will ever be compliant.

Fed up

Tired of or frustrated with something or someone.

The doctor was fed up with the patient not taking his medications as prescribed.

Fed up to the gills *or* Fed up to the teeth

Tired of or frustrated with something or someone.

The doctor was fed up to the gills with the patient not taking his warnings about smoking seriously.

Feel dragged out

To feel exhausted.

Halfway through her physical therapy session, the patient complained that she felt dragged out, so the therapist told her to stop and get some rest.

Feel fit

To feel healthy.

The patient reported feeling fit since she started taking yoga classes twice a week.

Feel free

To be allowed or permitted to do something.

The doctor instructed the patient to feel free to take Tylenol as needed for her headaches.

Feel like a million dollars *or* Feel like a million bucks

To feel well-rested or refreshed.

At her post surgery follow-up visit, Liza told Dr. Franks that she felt like a million dollars.

Feel out of place

To be uncomfortable in a situation.

As the only male nurse at the hospital, Bob often felt out of place at staff meetings.

Feel (someone) out

To attempt to determine someone's thoughts or plans.

The doctor tried to feel the patient out to determine whether he actually wanted to go through with the surgery.

Feel up to (something)

To feel well enough or prepared enough to do something.

Hopefully, the patient will feel up to getting out of bed tomorrow.

Fence (someone) in

To restrict someone's movements or actions.

David felt fenced in in the small hospital room.

Fend for (oneself)

To care for oneself without assistance from anyone else.

Even though Jeanie must adjust to getting around in a wheelchair, she is confident that she'll soon be able to fend for herself.

Few and far between

Rare.

The hours that the patient felt pain-free were few and far between.

Fiddle while Rome burns

To do nothing while something disastrous happens.

The resident just fiddled while Rome burned, and the patient, who needed immediate attention, didn't receive care until the doctor arrived.

Fight against time

To hurry to meet a deadline or to do something quickly.

The doctors fought against time to get the patient to the operating room without delay.

Fight (someone) tooth and nail

To struggle against someone or something with great determination.

The patient fought the orderlies tooth and nail when they tried to restrain him.

Fighting chance

A good possibility of success.

The chemotherapy gave the patient a fighting chance against the aggressive cancer.

Figure on (something)

To expect something.

We figure on at least 100 MTs being certified by the end of the year.

Fill (someone) in

To inform someone of something.

The doctor asked the nurse to fill him in on the details of the patient's care.

Fill (someone's) shoes

Take the place of some other person.

Ian is such a hard worker that it will be hard to fill his shoes when he leaves.

Fill (something) to the brim

To fill something all the way to the top of the container.

The antihistamine left the patient very thirsty, so he asked the nurse to fill his water glass to the brim.

Final fling

The last act of enjoyment before a big change.

Before his gastric bypass surgery, the patient decided to have one final fling and went to dinner with his friends.

Finders keepers

An expression implying that anything one finds automatically belongs to them; part of the phrase "finders keepers, losers weepers."

When Marla found a dollar bill on the floor, she cried, "Finders keepers!" and picked it up.

Find it in (one's) heart

To feel compassion.

The hospital needed volunteers and hoped that some members of the community would find it in their hearts to help out.

Find (one's) way

To discover the path or route; to be able to move about an area with confidence.

After a week of residency, Jeff has no trouble finding his way around the hospital.

Find out

To discover facts.

When Janet found out she was pregnant, she immediately started preparing for motherhood.

Find out the hard way

To learn something by experience, especially by unpleasant experience.

The patient found out the hard way that not taking her medications as instructed caused her to get worse instead of better.

Fine and dandy

All right.

The patient said she was feeling fine and dandy and had no immediate problems.

Fine kettle of fish

An unsatisfactory situation.

There are four hours of dictation to complete and the system is down: This is a fine kettle of fish we're in!

Fire away

To begin to talk rapidly or ask a series of questions.

The patient fired away with many questions about his condition.

Fire on all cylinders

Working at full strength and capacity.

Irene knew she needed to get a good night's sleep if she wanted to fire on all cylinders.

First and foremost

Most importantly.

First and foremost, you need to study for tomorrow's test.

First come, first served

Service given in order of arrival.

The hospital emergency room doctors see patients on a first come, first served basis.

First of all

Before proceeding.

First of all, let's get your medical history, and then the doctor will perform the physical.

First thing

Before anything else.

We will test Jan's blood sugar first thing in the morning.

Fish for (something)

To try to get something in a sneaky way; often refers to information, answers, or compliments.

The patient spent quite a bit of time asking the nurse questions, fishing for more information on the doctor's plans for treatment.

Fish or cut bait

Either do the job one is supposed to do or quit.

Tony gave the drug one more chance, but he told the doctor he was ready to fish or cut bait.

Fit in

To be comfortable within a group.

It took some time for the new nurse to fit in with the rest of the staff.

Fit like a glove

The perfect size.

The uniform fit like a glove.

Fit (someone or something) in

To make time to see someone or do something.

Rachel called her optometrist to see if he could fit her in for an afternoon appointment.

Fit (someone) to a T

To suit a person very well.

Seth's new job in the pediatric wing fit his youthful personality to a T.

Fit to be tied

Very angry or upset.

Robert was fit to be tied when the doctor called at the last minute and cancelled his appointment.

Fix (someone's) wagon

To punish someone; to get even.

Trevor took credit for my idea, so I'll have to fix his wagon.

Fizzle out

To come to a stop gradually.

After a few days, the patient's enthusiasm for the new brace fizzled out.

Flat as a pancake

A very level surface.

Bobby smashed the can flat as a pancake.

Flat broke

With no money at all.

Jessica is flat broke and can't even afford the $10 co-pay for her doctor's appointment.

Flat out

In a straightforward manner.

The nurse told the patient flat out to change his attitude.

Flesh and blood

A living human body; *also*, an immediate family member.

The therapist reminded Clarence that he was only flesh and blood, and there were limits to his abilities.

The elderly patient was happy to know he would be living with his own flesh and blood rather than being sent to a nursing home.

Flight of fancy

An idea or suggestion that is out of touch with reality.

The psychologist reported that the patient had flights of fancy about being elected president.

Flip (one's) lid

To suddenly become angry, crazy, or enthusiastic.

The nurse flipped her lid when the patient removed his own IV.

Flunk out

To fail a course in school.

Debbie missed so many classes when she was sick that she ended up flunking out of pre-med school.

Fly-by-night

Irresponsible; untrustworthy.

Dr. Lawrence didn't expect Juan to get much out of rehab because he approached it in a fly-by-night manner.

Fly off the handle

To lose one's temper.

Dr. Cho learned to control his temper and not to fly off the handle in front of his patients.

Follow suit

To mimic another's actions.

When he saw how much weight loss success his wife

achieved following her exercise program, Jack followed suit and began jogging three times a week.

Food for thought

Something to consider.

Whether or not they objected to the moral implications, the doctors all agreed that the lecture on stem cell research offered good food for thought.

Fool around

To play with someone or something.

The doctor warned Hal not to fool around with prescription drugs and to always follow the dosage instructions carefully.

Foot the bill

To pay for something.

Because Adam's injury occurred on hospital property, the hospital was footing the bill for his treatment.

Footloose and fancy-free

Without responsibilities, commitments, or worries.

Despite being confined to a wheelchair, Amy always seemed footloose and fancy-free.

For all intents and purposes

Almost; virtually.

She still sneezes occasionally, but for all intents and purposes, Rosie has recovered from her cold.

For all (one) cares

Of no consequence to someone.

Dr. Sokolov told Chelsea that, for all he cared, she could skip getting a flu shot.

For all (one) knows

Based on one's limited knowledge of something.

For all I know, Mrs. Garza may have already left to go home.

For chicken feed

For little or nothing.

Cameron got the drug for chicken feed by choosing the generic instead of the name brand.

For days on end

Continuously; without end.

The patient complained of pain for days on end.

For fear of (something)

In the event that something unpleasant occurs.

Alan didn't want to see the doctor for fear of his flu-like symptoms actually being a more serious illness.

For good

Permanently.

Although the medication did not work, the surgery should fix the problem for good.

For good measure

Just in case; as an extra step.

Manuel feels fine on his present regimen, but Dr. Patel added aspirin for good measure.

For kicks

For fun.

For kicks, Ann and Brent planned to play a practical joke on the other nurses.

For openers

First.

The conference should be very interesting; for openers, Dr. Altman will speak on current trends in gastroenterology.

For peanuts

For little or nothing.

People often think that doctors make a lot of money, but when they start their medical careers, they usually work for peanuts.

For real

Genuine.

The new drug was so effective and had so few side effects that the researchers could hardly believe it was for real.

For that matter

In addition to; along the same lines.

The patient constantly argues with Dr. McCall's recommendations, and for that matter, so does his wife.

For the asking

Readily available.

The anesthesiologist provided epidurals for the asking to women whose labor pain became unbearable.

For the best

Good despite the way it may seem.

The patient's condition deteriorated rapidly and he passed away, but it was all for the best. He would have never recovered fully from the extensive injuries.

For the birds

Worthless; undesirable.

The patient felt that the therapy was for the birds since it did not improve his symptoms.

For the life of (someone)

Despite every attempt.

For the life of me, I can't seem to recall the doctor's name.

For the moment

At the present time.

The patient is stable for the moment, but the nursing staff will monitor her closely overnight.

For the most part

In general.

For the most part, Ronald follows a very healthy lifestyle.

For the record

To state publicly.

For the record, I always comply with prescribed treatments.

For the sake of (someone or something)

In someone or something's best interest.

Congress passed HIPAA regulations for the sake of patient privacy.

For the taking

Readily available.

At the medical convention, the pharmaceutical company had samples of its new antihistamine for the taking.

Forbidden fruit

Something that someone is not allowed to have or participate in.

The nutritionist told Lester that if he wanted to lose weight, fried foods were forbidden fruit.

Force (someone's) hand

To coerce a person to reveal plans, strategies, or secrets.

Mr. Milo refused to tell the doctor what supple-

ments he had been taking, so the doctor had to force his hand to obtain the necessary information.

Force to be reckoned with

An important or intimidating person or situation.

The FDA is a force to be reckoned with for many pharmaceutical companies.

Fore and aft

At the front and the back.

The patient felt a draft from fore and aft because his hospital gown was not closed all the way.

Forever and a day

For an extremely long time.

The patient felt like he would be on his medications forever and a day.

Forever and ever

For eternity.

After 24 hours on call, the resident felt like he had been on his feet forever and ever.

Forgive and forget

To make amends and move past a disagreement.

When the doctor's treatment protocol relieved her arthritis pain, Maureen decided to forgive and forget his rude comments.

Fork money out

To pay for something.

Kimberly was reluctant to fork money out for another x-ray because she had already had one the week before.

Fork (something) over

To give something to someone.

If the patient refuses to fork over the signed consent forms, then we'll have to cancel the procedure.

Form an opinion

To take a stance.

The doctor needed to see more clinical research to form an opinion on the new drug.

Forty winks

A short nap.

The patient tried to catch forty winks while waiting for the doctor to examine his x-rays.

Foul play

Illegal activity; bad practices.

The patient's lacerations indicated foul play, not an accident.

Foul up

A mistake.

Any foul up in healthcare can put people's lives in danger.

Free and clear

Without any additional obligation or responsibility.

The patient was discharged from the hospital free and clear.

Free-for-all

A disorganized event involving many people.

It was a free-for-all when the pharmaceutical company sponsored a no-charge health clinic at the mall.

Friend or foe

An ally or an enemy.

It is sometimes difficult for patients with an altered mental status to differentiate between friend or foe.

Frightened out of (one's) wits

To be very scared.

The sound of the MRI frightened Dorothy out of her wits.

From day to day

On a regular basis.

The patient must check her glucose level from day to day.

From door to door

To visit all the houses or buildings on a street.

Jodi went from door to door collecting donations to

purchase medical supplies for Third World countries.

From near and far

Both close in proximity and from great distances.

People came from near and far to be seen at the world-renowned cancer clinic.

From start to finish

From the beginning to the end.

The nurse will monitor Mike throughout his hospital stay, from start to finish, to ensure that he follows the doctor's orders.

From the bottom of (one's) heart

Sincerely.

The patient thanked the hospital staff from the bottom of her heart for giving her such good care.

From the cradle to the grave

From birth to death.

The new electronic patient record will follow you from the cradle to the grave.

From the ground up

Starting with nothing.

We must develop the alternative medicine training program from the ground up.

From the outset

From the beginning.

Walt had problems with the medication's side effects from the outset.

From the word go

From the beginning.

The patient was enthusiastic about his therapy from the word go.

From time to time

Occasionally.

Edward will return from time to time to have his cholesterol checked.

From way back

From far in the past.

Dr. Zane knew the patient from way back; they went to college together.

Full of beans

Incorrect, dishonest, or silly.

Jamey thought his doctor was full of beans to recommend acupuncture.

Full steam ahead

Quickly and energetically.

The contractors moved full steam ahead to build the much-needed hospital addition.

Fun and games

Worthless or lighthearted things.

Sometimes teenagers don't take their own health seriously enough and think that it is all fun and games.

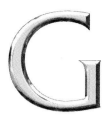

G

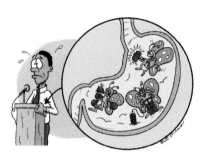

*Get butterflies
in your stomach*

Gain ground

To make progress.

The doctor was pleased to see that the patient was gaining ground.

Gang up

To form into a group and attack someone.

The drug addict felt everyone ganged up on him during the intervention.

Gear up

To prepare for something.

The surgeon geared up for the lengthy quadruple bypass procedure.

Generous to a fault

Too giving.

Dr. Nils is always giving free medical care to those who can't afford it. He is generous to a fault.

Get a bee in (one's) bonnet

To have an idea or a thought that remains in one's mind.

The therapist got a bee in her bonnet to use hypnosis to help Renee quit smoking.

Get a big send off

To have a celebration before departing.

After many weeks of being in the hospital, the patient got a big send off from the nursing staff when he was finally discharged.

Get a break

To have good fortune.

With all of her other health problems, Adele felt that she got a break when her blood test for diabetes came back negative.

Get a bright idea

To have a clever thought.

As he set the boy's broken arm in a cast, the doctor

warned him not to get any more bright ideas like skateboarding down the steps.

Get a charge out of (someone or something)

To receive special pleasure or amusement from something or someone.

The patient got a charge out of Julius, the physical therapist, especially when he tried to demonstrate the Thera-Band.

Get a charley horse

To develop a cramp in the arm or leg.

If you stretch in the wrong direction, you may get a charley horse in your leg.

Get a checkup

To have a physical exam.

Susie has an appointment with Dr. Mancini to get a checkup tomorrow.

Get a clean bill of health

To be pronounced in excellent physical condition.

The patient got a clean bill of health from his doctor.

Get a dirty look from (someone)

To receive an unpleasant facial expression from someone.

The doctor gave Stan a dirty look when he admitted that he was still smoking.

Get a free hand

To be granted complete control.

The dietician got a free hand in creating the patient's new diet regimen.

Get a frog in (one's) throat

To temporarily speak in a raspy or altered voice.

Wendi got a frog in her throat this morning and had difficulty making her presentation to the hospital board of directors.

Get a grasp of (something)

To understand something.

The new nurse had a hard time getting a grasp of the hospital's regulations.

Get a handle on (something)

To understand something.

Kristian finally got a handle on the medical terms he was studying.

Get a head start

To begin something sooner than anyone else.

The x-ray technician set up her first appointment at 7 a.m. because she wanted to get a head start on the busy day.

Get a jump-start on (something or someone)

To take the initiative and begin something.

Although he was still an undergraduate student,

Erik took an internship at the local hospital to get a jump-start on his medical career.

Get a life

To find some purpose for existing.

The doctor told the patient to get a life and stop spending so much time at work.

Get a load of (someone or something)

Look at someone or something.

Get a load of Jenny's new outfit.

Get a rain check

To make a request to postpone something or to take advantage of an opportunity at a later date.

I'm not feeling very well, so can I get a rain check on tonight's dinner plans?

Get a raw deal

To receive unfair or bad treatment.

Brad got a raw deal on his medication because he had to pay full price even though it was listed on the insurance company's drug formulary.

Get a reputation

To be recognized because of a particular characteristic.

After 20 years at her job, Stella got a reputation as an expert in the MT industry.

Get a rise out of (someone)

To elicit a response from someone, usually anger or laughter.

The psychiatrist tried to get a rise out of Carrie to determine what would trigger her anger.

Get a rough idea

To get a general sense about something or someone.

The doctor wanted the patient to walk every other day to get a rough idea of his exercise tolerance.

Get a run for (one's) money

To be challenged by someone or something.

Considering the 3-hour interview process, the prospective medical students certainly got a run for their money from the university admissions committee.

Get a slap on the wrist

To receive a light punishment.

Jeff only got a slap on the wrist for not checking in on his patients as often as he should have.

Get a taste of (one's) own medicine

To experience similar circumstances to those one has caused others to experience.

Dr. Orwell got a taste of his own medicine when his cardiologist told him to cut down on his salt intake.

Get a tongue-lashing

To receive a severe scolding.

The patient got a tongue-lashing from the doctor for not taking his medications properly.

Get a word in edgewise

To manage to say something.

Brooke could not get a word in edgewise because Shannon and Karen were talking so much.

Get all dolled up

To pay special attention to one's appearance.

The nurse helped Mrs. Horton get all dolled up for her family's visit.

Get along in years

To grow older.

The patient was getting along in years and would soon need assisted care.

Get along on a shoestring

To live on very little money.

The doctor was careful what medications he prescribed because the patient was just getting along on a shoestring.

Get ants in (one's) pants

To become nervous and agitated.

The toddler was jumping around like he had ants in his pants!

Get around

To navigate or to be experienced; *also,* to evade.

Jack has lived here for many years and really knows how to get around the city.

The patient tried to get around answering direct questions, hoping her doctor wouldn't discover how sick she really was.

Get around to (something)

To find time to do something.

The doctor said he would try to get around to completing his past-due dictations this afternoon.

Get away from it all

To take a break from one's daily or work routine.

The doctor recommended that Mr. Ackerman get away from it all and go on a short vacation to gain back some of his lost energy.

Get away with (something)

To do something wrong and not get punished for it.

Sharon tried to cheat on the test, but she did not get away with it.

Get back at (someone)

To exact revenge on someone.

The patient wanted to get back at his wife for having him admitted to the rehabilitation clinic.

Get back into circulation

To resume social activities and interaction.

After hospitalization, the patient gradually tried to get back into circulation by making dinner plans with his friends once a week.

Get back on (one's) feet

To recover and become independent again.

It took Adam a while to get back on his feet after the accident.

Get better

To improve.

The patient started to get better after his treatment.

Get busy

To start working.

When Beth finally got busy, she finished her rounds in no time.

Get butterflies in (one's) stomach

To feel nervous.

The patient had butterflies in her stomach before surgery.

Get by

To remain productive with very limited resources.

Despite the department's inadequate supply of reference books, the staff manages to get by on the volumes they do have.

Get carried away

To be overcome with emotion.

Sometimes patients' families get carried away during a crisis.

Get cold feet

To become fearful of something.

The patient scheduled his surgery for the very next day because he feared he would get cold feet if he waited too long.

Get credit

Receive praise or acknowledgment.

The nurse got credit for saving the patient's life.

Get down to business

To begin.

The hospital administrator wanted to get down to business and work on the budget.

Get down to the nitty-gritty

To discuss only the facts.

Rather than engaging in small talk, Dr. Green always gets down to the nitty-gritty with his patients right away.

Get goose bumps

For one's skin to feel prickly or become bumpy due to fear, excitement, or cold temperatures.

Patients often get goose bumps before a procedure.

Get in on (something)

To become involved with something.

The cardiologist and the gastroenterologist both wanted to get in on the treatment plans for the patient.

Get into a jam

To encounter difficulty.

Nancy took on too many responsibilities at once and got herself into a jam.

Get into full swing

To move into the peak of activity.

The nursing station gets into full swing by mid morning.

Get into hot water

To encounter trouble or difficulty due to one's own actions.

If a patient pushes rehab too hard, he could get into hot water.

Get it

To receive punishment or a lecture; *also,* to fully understand something.

The patient refused to take his medication and is going to get it from the doctor.

Get nowhere fast

To make no progress.

Without adequate staffing, the extended rehab program got nowhere fast.

Get off it

Don't talk nonsense.

Get off it; you don't know what you are talking about.

Get off on the wrong foot

To start something badly.

The patient and the doctor got off on the wrong foot from the beginning when they disagreed about the severity of his condition.

Get off (someone's) back

Leave someone alone.

Justin told his friend to get off his back about exercising more.

Get off the hook

To be excused from an obligation.

I didn't have time to attend the lecture, so Austin helped me get off the hook.

Get off to a flying start

To have a very successful beginning.

Dr. Smith's new practice got off to a flying start, with a full patient load on his first day.

Get (one's) act together

To become focused or organized.

Travis needs to get his act together and take rehab seriously.

Get (one's) ducks in a row

To become organized.

Lena can end her shift as soon as she gets her ducks in a row and files all her paperwork.

Get (one's) feet wet

To gain experience in something.

The new MTs are just getting their feet wet.

Get (one's) foot in the door

To make oneself known.

If I can get my foot in the door at the hospital, I think I can get one of the open resident positions.

Get (one's) head above water

To begin to overcome one's problems.

If Ewan follows a budget, he will be able to get his head above water sooner.

Get (one's) just desserts

To experience a negative end result after one has caused problems.

Alexandra got her just desserts for cheating on her final exam when she didn't graduate from nursing school with the rest of her class.

Get (one's) money's worth

To be satisfied with a purchase or the amount of money spent on something.

Sue's nutritionist gave her a comprehensive meal plan to follow for the entire year, so Sue felt as though she got her money's worth for the session.

Get (one's) wires crossed

To be confused about something.

The patient must have gotten his wires crossed because he showed up on the wrong day for his appointment.

Get on (someone's) nerves

To irritate someone.

After several days, the two patients sharing room 343 got on each other's nerves.

Get physical

To use physical force against someone.

The nursing staff had to get physical to restrain the combative patient.

Get rolling

To get started.

Mick needs to get rolling with his occupational therapy program if he ever wants to recover.

Get (someone) out of a jam

To help someone resolve a problem or bad situation.

Gabriella changed shifts with me to get me out of a jam.

Get (someone's) number

To discover someone's true motives.

Professor Benedict wondered why Adrienne always offered to help him with his paperwork, but he got her number when he caught her cheating on the exam.

Get (something) across to (someone)

To convey information to someone.

The nurse tried to get it across to Patrick that he had to take his medication on time.

Get (something) into (someone's) thick head *or* Get (something) into (someone's) thick skull

To manage to make someone understand something.

The nurse had a difficult time getting the visitation policy into the patient's mother's thick head.

Get (something) off the ground

To start something.

It took four years to raise enough funds to get construction of the children's hospital off the ground.

Get (something) out of (one's) system

To discuss or do something that one has been thinking about for some time.

Dr. Moore encouraged his patients to get things out of their system by keeping a journal.

Get (something) out in the open

To confess something.

The therapist encouraged the patient to get her fears out in the open.

Get (something) straight

To understand something clearly.

The discharge nurse reviewed the orders with the patient one last time to make sure that he got them straight.

Get (something) together

To organize something.

Dr. Jimenez got his recommendations together and went over each of them in detail with the patient.

Get (something) under way

To start something.

The patient was transferred out of the ER to get treatment under way.

Get the ball rolling

To start something.

The doctor got the ball rolling by scheduling the patient's therapy sessions.

Get the boot

To be sent away or dismissed.

The intern got the boot after he misplaced the doctor's files.

Get the brush-off

To be ignored.

Maryann thought the insurance company would help her, but she got the brush-off from the representative.

Get the feel of (something)

To learn the way something works.

It only took the patient a week to get the feel of his new prosthesis.

Get the go-ahead

To receive approval to begin or continue something.

We will continue the patient's treatment once we get the go-ahead from the insurance company.

Get the hang of (something)

To learn how to do something.

The resident got the hang of giving injections right away.

Get the runaround

To encounter a series of excuses and delays.

I have been trying to schedule my annual checkup

for an hour, but I keep getting the runaround from the clinic receptionist.

Get to the bottom of (something)

To determine the cause of something.

The doctor questioned Anika thoroughly, trying to get to the bottom of her symptoms.

Get to the heart of the matter

To determine the cause of a problem.

Dr. Massari interviewed the patient extensively about her symptoms, trying to get to the heart of the matter.

Get to the point

To arrive at the important part of a conversation.

Dr. Horton waited patiently for Ms. Abbott to get to the point of her story.

Get tough

Become firm with someone.

The doctor had to get tough with the resident after he neglected to follow proper procedure for the third time.

Get-up-and-go

Energy.

Hopefully the new medication will counteract the patient's lethargy and give him some get-up-and-go.

Get up on the wrong side of the bed

To be in a bad mood.

Caleb yelled at the nurse, so she assumed that he got up on the wrong side of the bed.

Get wind of (something)

To hear about something.

Every time Sarah gets wind of a new pharmaceutical drug, she asks her doctor to prescribe it to her.

Get worked up

To get excited or emotionally distressed about something.

The doctor wanted the patient to undergo stress management because he gets worked up so easily.

Ghost of a chance

A very slight possibility.

Dr. Phillips doesn't think there's a ghost of a chance that the new protocol will work.

Give-and-take

Willingness to compromise.

For doctors and nurses to work effectively together in emergency situations, it requires give-and-take.

Give (someone) a break

To be less strict or severe with someone.

Even though he hadn't made much progress, the

physical therapist knew Carl had tried his best, so she gave him a break and didn't reprimand him.

Give (someone) a hard time

To tease someone; to give someone unnecessary difficulty.

The doctor gave the patient a hard time about going off his diet.

Give (someone) the benefit of the doubt

To make a judgment in someone's favor when the evidence is neither for nor against the person.

Because she had never been in trouble before, Brittany's supervisor gave her the benefit of the doubt.

Give (someone) the go-ahead

To extend permission for something to begin.

The doctor gave Salvatore the go-ahead to begin treatment.

Give (someone) the green light

To extend permission for something to begin.

The doctor gave the patient the green light to start speech therapy.

Give (someone) the once-over

To quickly examine someone visually; to look at someone with interest.

Dr. Barton gave Martin the once-over before sur-

gery and confirmed that all his vital signs were normal.

Give (someone) the third degree

To extensively question someone in great detail.

The patient felt uncomfortable after the therapist gave her the third degree during their first session.

Give (something) a lick and a promise

To do something quickly and poorly.

The ER was so busy the cleaning crew could only give it a lick and a promise until the shift ended.

Given to understand

Led to believe.

Dr. Christianson had been given to understand that his assistant finished dictating his charts, and he became angry when he found out otherwise.

Go against the grain

To deviate from the established method or popular opinion.

Bess decided to go against the grain and chose to treat her cancer with herbal therapies instead of chemotherapy.

Go away empty handed

To depart with nothing.

The clinic offers informational pamphlets and free

samples of certain medicines, so patients never go away empty handed.

Go by the book

To follow the rules or established protocol exactly.

Dr. Hernandez never considers complementary and alternative medicine when treating his patients: He goes by the book and only prescribes conventional therapies.

Go cold turkey

To stop abruptly.

After 20 years of smoking, Marissa decided to go cold turkey and quit once and for all.

Go downhill

To decline.

The patient began to go downhill around midnight and expired at 1 a.m.

Go Dutch

To pay for one's own expenses.

Shenae thought she and Kevin would go Dutch on their date, but he offered to pay for her movie ticket.

Go fifty-fifty

To divide the cost of something in half with someone.

Peggy and Michele will go fifty-fifty on the cost of the hotel room.

Go from bad to worse

To progressively deteriorate.

The patient went from bad to worse when her sinus infection developed into pneumonia.

Go hog-wild

To overindulge or behave crazily.

Scott ate a few holiday sweets at the party, but based on his doctor's diet advice, he didn't go hog-wild.

Go into effect

To become active.

The new Medicare prescription drug coverage will go into effect later this year.

Go it alone

To do something by oneself.

After much thought, the patient decided to go it alone and did not involve his family in planning his future treatment.

Go off half-cocked

To speak or act hastily and without thinking it through.

It can be dangerous to go off half-cocked with a new exercise regimen without meeting with a doctor first.

Go off on a tangent

To lecture angrily.

When the nursing staff does not follow his orders exactly, Dr. Miller goes off on a tangent.

Go on a binge

To do too much of something.

After going on a binge with alcohol, Andre checked himself into rehab.

Go on a fishing expedition

To attempt to uncover information.

Ted refused to be forthcoming with details of his family history, so his psychologist had to go on a fishing expedition to learn more.

Go on and on

To continue infinitely.

The patient could go on and on about her numerous health problems.

Go over like a lead balloon

To meet with disapproval or displeasure.

Dr. Linden's suggestion to eliminate red meat went over like a lead balloon with Mr. Lowry.

Go over (someone's) head

To be beyond one's understanding; *also,* to bypass someone with less authority so one can address someone who has greater authority.

The doctor's instructions tend to be very complicated and usually go over his patients' heads.

Go over (something) with a fine-tooth comb

To examine something very carefully.

The doctor reviewed the patient's chart with a fine-tooth comb but found nothing out of the ordinary.

Go sky high

To increase exponentially.

Without healthcare reform, experts expect insurance premiums to go sky high over the next few years.

Go stir crazy

To become anxious due to confinement.

Meredith knew she would go stir crazy if her obstetrician recommended complete bed rest for the last trimester of her pregnancy.

Go the distance

To complete something.

The patient was able to go the distance with his chemotherapy.

Go through the change

To experience menopause.

Beverly often complains to her husband about the frequent night sweats and hot flashes that occur as she goes through the change.

Go through the motions

To make a feeble effort to do something.

The patient complained of feeling fatigued to the point of barely being able to care for herself. She was just going through the motions.

Go through the proper channels

To follow the correct procedures.

The patient had to go through the proper channels to get his insurance claim approved.

Go to any length

To do whatever is necessary.

Simon will go to any length to help his sister beat her chemical dependency.

Go to pieces

To have an emotional breakdown.

The patient went to pieces after she heard her prognosis.

Go too far

To do more than is acceptable.

The nutritionist worried that, with Holly's history of anorexia, she would go too far in limiting her food intake.

Go under the knife

To have a surgical procedure done.

The patient preferred not to go under the knife without trying noninvasive therapies first.

Go whole hog

To be extravagant.

The night before she started her low-carbohydrate diet, Emma decided to go whole hog and ordered every dessert on the menu.

Goes to show

Proves a point.

Yvette has lost 30 pounds! That just goes to show you what dedication and a healthy lifestyle will do.

Gold mine of information

Someone or something that can provide a great deal of information.

Bonnie is a gold mine of information about current medical transcription practices.

Good for nothing

Someone or something without value.

Gwen thought medical school had been good for nothing as far as actually preparing her to deal with difficult patients.

Gray area

An undefined matter.

The procedure's outcome was still a gray area, so the doctor could not assure the patient's family of success.

Greatest thing since sliced bread

The best thing there ever was.

The new drug worked so well to relieve Quincy's migraines that he told his doctor it was the greatest thing since sliced bread.

Greek to (someone)

Unintelligible.

Ned told the doctor that the diagnosis was all Greek to him, so she arranged for him to receive additional information that would help him better understand his health issues.

Green around the gills

To look sickly.

Pete ate too much pizza last night, and this morning he looks a little green around the gills.

Green with envy

Jealous.

When the doctor praised Fiona's presence of mind, the other nurses were green with envy.

Gross (someone) out

To disgust someone.

Observing surgery for the first time can gross medical students out.

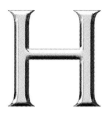

H

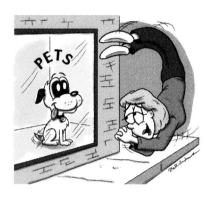

Head over heels

Hacked off

Mad or angry.

Mr. Mavros was hacked off after waiting so long to see the doctor.

Had better (do something)

Should or ought to do something.

The doctor had better do something quick, before the patient gets any worse.

Hale and hearty

Very healthy.

Since Mark appeared to be hale and hearty during

the initial exam, he didn't need any additional followup testing.

Halfhearted

Unenthusiastic.

Angelique made only a halfhearted attempt to improve during her therapy sessions.

Hammer (something) out

To work hard to reach an agreement.

The lawyers sat down to hammer out the contract.

Handle with kid gloves

To be very careful with a person or situation.

The ER staff had to handle the frightened child with kid gloves.

Hang(ing) by a thread

To be in an uncertain position.

After sustaining numerous injuries, the accident victim was hanging on by a thread.

Hang loose

To relax.

After work, everyone wanted to hang loose and watch a movie.

Hang out

To spend time somewhere.

Everyone went to Joe's to hang out for the evening.

Hard-and-fast

Rigid, especially when applied to rules, laws, or regulations.

The hospital has a hard-and-fast rule about breaching patient confidentiality.

Hard nut to crack

Difficult person or thing to deal with.

Though we've run just about every available test, this is really a hard nut to crack. We're still unable to determine what is causing the patient's symptoms.

Have a bone to pick (with someone)

To have a matter to discuss with someone.

The doctor had a bone to pick with the physical therapist because he did not do all the patient's exercises as ordered.

Have a change of heart

To change one's attitude or decision.

Kelly had a change of heart about which treatment she preferred after she learned all the facts.

Have a chip on (one's) shoulder

To portray an angry or resentful demeanor.

Michael always argues with the nurses, so they feel he has a chip on his shoulder.

Have a clear conscience

To be free of guilt.

The emergency department staff had a clear conscious, since they did everything they could to try and save the patient.

Have a good command of (something)

To know something well.

Medical transcriptionists need to have a good command of English grammar and punctuation.

Have a good thing going

To have a beneficial arrangement or situation.

Chris has a good thing going, since his schedule allows him to work two jobs without conflict.

Have a green thumb

To have the ability to grow plants well.

Trudy's beautiful rose garden is proof that she has quite a green thumb.

Have a heart of gold

To be generous and kind.

Stella has a heart of gold; she would do anything for anyone.

Have a rough time

To experience a difficult period.

Since his wife's death, Mr. Schaffer has been having a rough time and needs someone to look after him.

Have a screw loose

To act silly or crazy.

John always plays jokes on his friends. Sometimes they think he has a screw loose.

Have a spaz

To get visibly and demonstrably angry. *[slang]*

The patient would have a spaz if the nurse didn't bring her medications on time.

Have a stroke

To get visibly and demonstrably angry. *[slang]*

I thought Dr. Harris would have a stroke, he was so mad.

Have a thing about (someone or something)

To feel strongly about someone or something.

Naomi has a thing about the beach; she just hates the sand.

Have a whale of a time

To have an exciting time.

We had a whale of a time at the baseball game.

Have an ax to grind

To have something to complain about.

The patient had an ax to grind with the insurance company when they denied his claim.

Have foot-in-mouth disease

To embarrass oneself through a silly verbal blunder.

Sally spoke out of turn, and Jim teased her that she must have foot-in-mouth disease.

Have (one's) cake and eat it too

To be able to take advantage of two seemingly contradictory things.

People often want to be healthier without giving up their bad habits, but you can't have your cake and eat it too.

Have (one's) heart set on (something)

To have intense hopes for something.

Dorothy had her heart set on having a baby girl, but she gave birth to a boy.

Have second thoughts about (someone or something)

To have doubts about someone or something.

After seeing a TV news program about botched facelifts, the patient had second thoughts about having cosmetic surgery.

Have (something) on the tip of (one's) tongue

To be on the verge of remembering a specific fact.

Just give me a minute; I have her name on the tip of my tongue.

Have the ball in (one's) court

To have control of a situation.

Now that William has been moved to the cardiac ward, the ball is in our court and we can provide him with the treatment he needs.

Have the Midas touch

To have a positive effect on everything one comes into contact with.

Rose's business is so successful. She certainly has the Midas touch.

Have to live with (something)

To have no other options.

The patient will have to live with his disabilities.

Head over heels

Deeply involved in a feeling or situation.

Mr. McFadden was head over heels in debt after his transplant.

High hopes

Elevated expectations for someone or something.

The drug company has high hopes for several of their drugs currently in clinical trials.

High man on the totem pole

The person at the top of a hierarchy.

I don't want to talk to just anyone; I want to see the high man on the totem pole.

High time

Almost overdue; about time.

It's high time the patient was taken for his tests.

Hit the road

To depart.

If we hit the road now, we will get to the show on time.

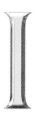

I

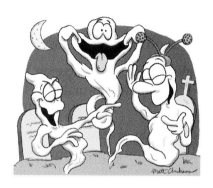

In good spirits

If push comes to shove

If a situation becomes difficult.

If push comes to shove, Mrs. Lake will be put on IV antibiotics to speed up the recovery process.

In all earnestness

Sincerely.

The doctor stressed in all earnestness the importance of staying on the prescribed regimen.

In all probability

Very likely.

In all probability, the patient will need to have surgery.

In any case

Regardless of what else may occur.

Hopefully the patient will be stronger tomorrow, but in any case, he will have to be discharged then.

In any event

Regardless of what else may occur.

In any event, the patient will undergo surgery this evening.

In bad sorts

In a bad mood.

Dr. Harnish could tell that the patient was in bad sorts when she didn't laugh at his jokes.

In brief

To be concise.

The doctor gave an overview, in brief, of the patient's condition.

In broad daylight

Publically visible.

Witnesses said that the shooting occurred in broad daylight.

In case

In the event that something takes place.

In case of an emergency, always carry your insurance card with you.

In concert

In cooperation.

The surgeons will treat the patient in concert to most effectively address the problem.

In earnest

Sincerely.

The patient promised, in earnest, to be very careful not to lift anything heavier than what the therapist advised.

In good hands

In the competent care of someone.

The patient is in good hands with the world-renowned vascular surgeon.

In good spirits

Happy and cheerful.

When the nurse told Hal he would be discharged the next day, it put him in good spirits.

In great demand

Wanted by many people.

The flu vaccine is in such great demand, the pharmaceutical company cannot keep up its supply.

In hopes of (something)

Expecting something.

Joy was in hopes of getting a raise.

In (just) a second

In a very short period of time.

I'll be there in just a second, but I need to take this call first.

In lieu of (something)

In place of something.

The patient chose treatment by medication in lieu of surgery.

In light of (something)

Because of certain knowledge.

In light of her test results, the doctor recommended that Jane undergo surgery.

In no time at all

Very quickly.

The nurse reassured the little boy that he would be home with his family and friends in no time at all.

In (one's) best interest

To one's advantage.

It is in your best interest to have a yearly physical exam.

In other words

Said in another, simpler way.

Dr. Wright told Don that he should eat nutritious foods and exercise regularly. In other words, he should start taking better care of himself.

In particular

Specifically, especially.

Sabrina couldn't say what was wrong, in particular; she just didn't feel good.

In progress

Happening now.

You can't go into the room; the test is already in progress.

In the doldrums

Sluggish, depressed.

Tony was in the doldrums today because the weather was rainy and gloomy.

In the flesh

In person.

We heard a famous cardiac surgeon was coming, in the flesh, to give a lecture.

In the hot seat

To be put in an uncomfortable situation.

The doctor put Brendan in the hot seat when he

began questioning him about his alcohol consumption.

In the nick of time

Just in time.

The EMS unit got to the accident scene in the nick of time.

In the prime of (one's) life

In the best and most productive period of life.

Jim is so physically fit and healthy that his doctor said he must be in the prime of his life.

It never rains, but it pours

Said when several bad things occur at the same time.

Johnny broke his arm the same day that Kristen broke her leg. Their mother couldn't help thinking that it never rains, but it pours.

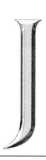

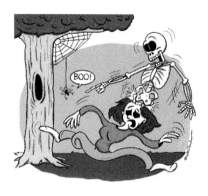

Jump out of your skin

Jack-of-all-trades

Someone who can do several different jobs as opposed to specializing in only one.

With his carpentry, plumbing, and painting skills, Martin is definitely a jack-of-all-trades.

Jazz (something) up

To make something more exciting.

Dr. Jones decided to jazz up his office by hanging some posters.

Jekyll and Hyde

Someone who appears to have both an evil and a good personality.

The patient shows signs of a Jekyll and Hyde personality.

Join forces

To combine resources to achieve a goal.

The neurological department and the surgery department will join forces in an effort to offer the patient the best mode of treatment.

Join the club

An expression indicating one person is in the same situation as the other.

You don't have any place to stay? Join the club - neither do we.

Joking aside

To be serious for a moment.

Joking aside, the situation could have been quite serious.

Judging by (something)

Considering something.

Judging by the way the MTs have been studying, I would say they are almost ready to take the certification exam.

Jump at the chance

To eagerly take advantage of an opportunity.

If I could travel around the world, I would jump at the chance.

Jump at the opportunity

To eagerly take advantage of an opportunity.

Paulette jumped at the opportunity to take the manager's position.

Jump to conclusions

To judge or decide something without having all the facts.

The doctor did not want to jump to conclusions about the diagnosis without further testing.

Jump the gun

To begin something too early.

Although he was anxious to begin treatment, Steve didn't want to jump the gun before learning all his options.

Just in case

In the event that something occurs.

Dr. Faulkner wanted to see the patient again in a week, just in case there were new developments.

Just what the doctor ordered

Exactly what is required, especially for health or comfort.

After a stressful week at work, Jennifer felt that a night on the town was just what the doctor ordered.

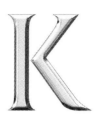

K

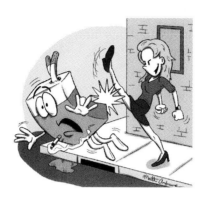

Kick the habit

Keel over

To fall down in a faint or in death.

The nurses had to support the weak patient because they were afraid he would keel over.

Keep a civil tongue

To speak decently and politely.

The patient was verbally combative and was reminded to keep a civil tongue.

Keep abreast of (something)

To stay informed.

The nurses kept the doctor abreast of the changes in the patient's condition.

Keep after (someone)

To remind a person to continue something.

The physical therapist had to keep after Jan to do all the repetitions as directed.

Keep an eye out

To be watchful for someone or something.

Ms. Rogers tends to wander the halls, so the nurses try to keep an eye out for her.

Keep at (something)

To continue doing something.

Dr. Brown urged the patient to keep at his attempts to quit smoking.

Keep company with

To spend a lot of time with certain individuals.

Mona's mother was concerned about the people she chose to keep company with.

Keep food down

To keep food in one's stomach, as opposed to vomiting.

The patient was given an antiemetic medication to help her keep food down.

Keep (one's) cool

Stay calm; hold one's temper.

Brad needs to learn to keep his cool in stressful situations.

Keep (one's) fingers crossed

To wish for good luck.

I am keeping my fingers crossed that your cholesterol test will show normal levels.

Keep on an even keel

To remain calm; to normalize or regulate someone or something.

The patient's antianxiety medications were increased to try to keep her on an even keel.

Keep pace

To move at the same speed.

For Toni, it was hard to keep pace with the rest of the class.

Keep (someone) down

To prevent someone from reaching their full potential.

Becca refused to let her husband's negative thinking keep her down.

Keep tabs

To monitor someone or something.

Ron's condition changed frequently, so the nurses had to keep tabs on him through the night.

Keep track of

To monitor, count, or stay informed of someone or something.

Between her heart medications, arthritis drugs, and blood thinners, Marge found it difficult to keep track of all her prescriptions.

Keep your shirt on!

Be patient.

You can use the phone when I'm finished. Until then, keep your shirt on!

Kick off

To start something, usually with a lot of flair and excitement.

The pharmaceutical company will kick off the promotional campaign for its new ACE inhibitor next month.

Kick the habit

To cease doing something.

Dave is a heavy smoker, but he is trying to kick the habit.

Kid around

To joke with someone.

The doctor had a great sense of humor and loved to kid around with his patients.

Kidding aside

To be serious for a moment.

Kidding aside, had the patient not come to the ER when she did, the situation would have been critical.

Kill two birds with one stone

To solve two problems with one solution.

If you get your prescription filled at the supermarket pharmacy, we can kill two birds with one stone and do our grocery shopping at the same time.

Knock-down, drag-out fight

A very serious fight.

The two teams got into a knock-down, drag-out fight and had to be separated.

Know-how

Knowledge and skill.

Scott has all the know-how to run a successful business.

Know the ropes

To know the various procedures involved in something.

Gary knows the ropes when it comes to creating new computer programs for dictation and transcription.

Knuckle down

To apply oneself wholeheartedly.

The patient really had to knuckle down in order to take control of her binge eating.

Knuckle under

To submit to someone or something.

The doctor cautioned Aaron that he would eventually have to knuckle under and be compliant with his medications if he wanted his condition to improve.

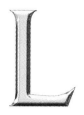

L

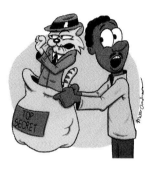

*Let the cat
out of the bag*

Labor of love

A task that one does simply for one's own satisfaction or pleasure.

The nurses enjoy their work in the NICU. It is a labor of love.

Laid-back

Relaxed.

Dr. Perez is very laid-back and always spends the first few minutes of an appointment simply chatting with his patients.

Laid off

To be placed out of work, sometimes temporarily.

Denise was laid off from her job and had to file for federal unemployment benefits.

Last-ditch effort

A final attempt.

As a last-ditch effort, the patient will undergo surgery.

Lay down the law

To state firmly what the rules are.

Noelle's doctor laid down the law about her not walking too soon on her leg.

Lay (someone) up

To cause someone to be ill in bed.

The cold laid Bruce up for a week.

Lay (something) on the line

Be honest and forthright.

The doctor laid it on the line when he told the patient he would need more therapy.

Lead (someone) down the garden path

To deceive someone.

Kathy was afraid the plastic surgeon was leading her down the garden path, and the surgery wouldn't produce the results promised.

Leaf through

To browse or thumb through printed material.

While he waited to see the doctor, Preston leafed through a pamphlet on privacy and security of his medical record.

Learn to live with (something)

To adapt to something unpleasant or painful.

Although he faced many challenges ahead, the patient would have to learn to live with his paralysis.

Leave a lot to be desired

To be lacking something important.

Gail thinks her doctor's brusque bedside manner leaves a lot to be desired.

Leave (oneself) wide open

To invite criticism or joking about oneself.

Without proper documentation of healthcare, the physician would leave himself wide open for a lawsuit.

Leave (someone) holding the bag

To let someone else take all the blame or responsibility for something.

The insurance company left Jasmine holding the bag when she did not report her emergency room visit within 48 hours.

Leave well enough alone

To let the situation remain as is; implies that any intervention may make the situation worse.

*John is making good progress, so we will leave well
enough alone for now.*

Let the cat out of the bag

To reveal a secret.

*Sean let the cat out of the bag that his wife was
pregnant.*

Lie down on the job

To do something poorly.

*The carpenter's sloppy work showed that he was
lying down on the job.*

Life of the party

A person who is lively and entertaining.

*With her great jokes and stories, Julie is always the
life of the party!*

Like a fish out of water

To be completely out of place.

*Pat felt like a fish out of water around the loud,
pushy people.*

Like apples and oranges

A comparison of two entities that are not similar.

The patient's last admission and this admission

cannot be compared; they are like apples and oranges.

Like clockwork

To progress with regularity and dependability.

Adam's physical therapy sessions went like clockwork, and he recovered very quickly.

Line of least resistance

The course of action that requires the least effort.

The doctor had to make simple, easy recommendations because the patient only wanted to take the line of least resistance.

Listen to reason

To yield to a reasonable opinion.

Even though they did not fully agree with the plan of treatment, the patient's family had to listen to reason and acknowledge its potential benefits.

Little by little

Slowly.

Little by little, the patient came around to accepting the diagnosis.

Live and let live

Not to interfere with other people's business.

Toby doesn't like it when people tell him what to do; he prefers to live and let live.

Live on borrowed time

To live longer than expected.

Vivian's doctor only gave her six months to live, so at this point, she is living on borrowed time.

Lock, stock, and barrel

Completely.

Greg has adopted every lifestyle change his doctor recommended, lock, stock, and barrel.

Look like the cat that swallowed the canary

To appear very smug and proud.

Dr. Olson is so proud of his patient's progress that he looks like the cat that swallowed the canary.

Lose face

To lose status and respect.

Adam is afraid of losing face among the other residents.

Lose heart

To become discouraged.

Miss Collins seemed to be losing heart, so the doctor tried to encourage her with stories of other patients who had successfully fought the disease.

Lose (one's) marbles

To become confused or crazy.

What is wrong with her? Has she lost her marbles?

Low man on the totem pole

The least important person.

Jesse felt like the low man on the totem pole when no one listened to his opinion.

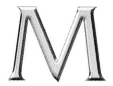

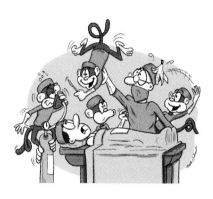

Monkey around

Mad as a hornet *or* Mad as a bee

Very angry.

Watch out, Joey is as mad as a hornet.

Mad enough to chew nails

Very angry.

When Dr. John realized his orders had not been followed, he was mad enough to chew nails.

Made for each other

A perfectly suited couple.

Tom and Susan were made for each other.

Made to order

Put together on request.

The course work was made to order, and includes sections on anatomy, pharmacology, and human disease processes.

Make a beeline for (someone or something)

To move straight towards someone or something.

After the 36-hour shift, the resident made a beeline for the hot shower.

Make a big deal about (something)

To have a strong reaction about something.

The therapist made a big deal about the patient's remarkable progress.

Make a clean breast of (something)

To confess; to tell all.

During drug rehab, Marty was urged to make a clean breast of all his mistakes.

Make a clean sweep

To completely clear out the old; also, to win by a large majority or to win a series of events.

A total hysterectomy was performed, making a clean sweep of the abdomen.

Make a dent in (something)

To make progress, usually on an overwhelming task.

I've just begun to make a dent in that pile of reports.

Make a fast buck

To make money with little effort.

Larry has trouble holding down a steady job because he is always out to make a fast buck.

Make a federal case of (something)

To exaggerate the seriousness of something.

Even though the billing conflict was resolved quickly, Olivia still called the hospital and made a federal case of it.

Make a living

How someone earns his or her livelihood.

The trainees were anxious to complete their course so they could begin to make a living at transcription.

Make a pitch for (something or someone)

To say something in support of someone or something.

Every year the hospital makes a pitch for additional funding for the oncology wing.

Make a point

To emphasize something.

The doctor always makes a point to check on his patients postoperatively to ensure they are stable and their vital signs are good.

Make a scene

To publicly cause a disturbance.

I know you're upset about the long wait to see the doctor, but there's no need to make a scene.

Make allowances for (someone or something)

To make special arrangements for someone or something.

In planning the patient's discharge, the doctor made allowances for home health care and physical therapy.

Make an all-out effort

To make a thorough and energetic attempt.

The patient made an all-out effort to improve during his speech therapy sessions.

Make an appointment

To schedule a meeting with someone.

The patient will make an appointment to see Dr. Fitzwilliam in one month's time.

Make good as (something) *or* Make good at (something)

To succeed at something.

Maryann wanted to make good as both a transcriptionist and a coder.

Make it up to (someone)

To repay someone; to a return favor.

Since Franklin worked Denise's weekend shift for her, she promised to make it up to him by buying him dinner.

Make light of (something)

To treat something as if it were unimportant or humorous.

Sometimes patients make light of their problems to help themselves feel better.

Make mincemeat out of (someone or something)

To beat up or overcome someone or something.

If you continue to bother Joey's little sister, he is going to find you and make mincemeat out of you.

Make or break (someone)

Lead to one's exaltation or ruin.

It is a difficult decision, and the resulting outcome will either make or break Dr. Witt's career.

Make points

To gain favor.

Rafi is trying to make points with Lillian by covering her shift in the emergency department.

Make sense (of something)

To understand.

The patient struggled to make sense of everything the physician told him about his condition.

Make (someone's) blood boil

To make someone very angry.

When John thinks about the injustices of the world, it makes his blood boil.

Make (someone's) blood run cold

To shock or terrify someone.

When Jake realized how serious the accident could have been, it made his blood run cold.

Make (something) from scratch

To make something starting with all the basic elements.

The patient baked Dr. Flegal a cake to express her gratitude for all he had done, but rather than using a mix, she made it from scratch.

Make the grade

To be satisfactory.

The professor told the med student that his test scores just did not make the grade.

Make up for lost time

To do much of something in very little time because of a late start or other delay.

Sasha missed classes for a week when she had the flu, and had to spend the entire weekend doing homework to make up for lost time.

Mark my words

Remember what I am saying.

You mark my words; this project will be successful!

Matter-of-fact

Businesslike; unfeeling.

Although he felt sad and frightened, Lee told his family about his cancer diagnosis in a matter-of-fact way.

Mealy mouthed

To speak in a manner that is indecisive or indirect.

Debbie was encouraged to speak her opinion openly and not be mealy mouthed.

Meat-and-potatoes

Basic, sturdy, and hearty.

Sam is a meat-and-potatoes kind of guy.

Melt in (one's) mouth

To taste very good.

Ellen's cake just melts in your mouth.

Middle-of-the-road

Halfway between two extremes.

When managing very different types of people, you can often create a more productive work environment by taking the middle-of-the-road approach.

Milestone

A very important event.

Being in remission for seven years is an important milestone for a breast cancer survivor.

Mind (one's) p's and q's

To mind one's manners.

Remember to mind your p's and q's when we are in the meeting with the hospital board of directors.

Monkey around

To be playful.

The students had a tendency to monkey around between periods rather than taking the time to get their work done.

Move heaven and earth to (do something)

To make a major effort to do something.

Shauna moved heaven and earth to get her son to the hospital after he fell out of the tree.

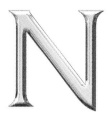

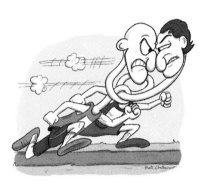

Neck and neck

Nail (something) down

To arrive at a firm and final decision.

Dr. Lu needed to consult with the other physicians before she could nail down a treatment plan for the patient.

Naked eye

The human eye, unassisted by optics.

The organism wasn't visible to the naked eye, but once it was under the microscope, the pathologist was able to classify it.

Near at hand

Close by.

The patient kept her nitroglycerin near at hand in case she began to have chest pain.

Neck and neck

Exactly even, especially in a race or a contest.

The class split up into teams, and the two groups were neck and neck in completing their projects.

Neither here nor there

Of no consequence or meaning.

The patient's wife had several theories on what was causing her husband's condition, but they were neither here nor there – what mattered was the doctor's diagnosis.

New ball game

A different set of circumstances.

Once the patient's tests results confirmed the doctor's suspicions, treating him became a new ball game.

New blood

New people in a group.

The hospital hired five new surgeons in an effort to introduce some new blood into the team.

Night on the town

A night of celebrating.

After a night on the town, the patient became seriously ill and was rushed to the hospital.

Nine-to-five job

A job with typical office hours, which are usually 9 a.m. until 5 p.m.

There aren't many nine-to-five jobs left! It seems we all work long hours.

No can do

Cannot do something.

Nick wanted to go to the movies rather than study, but Josh said, "No can do!"

No holds barred

With no restraints.

The patient can advance to full activities, no holds barred.

No ifs, ands, or buts

Absolutely no discussion or excuses.

According to the emergency department doctor, Damian needed an emergency appendectomy – no ifs, ands, or buts about it.

No news is good news

The assumption that all must be well if there is no information about someone or something.

Although the patient's family was waiting for some

word from the surgeon, they felt that no news was good news.

No skin off (one's) nose

Of no concern to someone.

It is no skin off my nose if you choose not to comply with the doctor's orders.

No skin off (one's) teeth

Of no concern to someone.

So what if the new equipment does not come in? It's no skin off your teeth.

No sooner said than done

Done quickly and obediently.

When the patient asked the nurse for water, it was no sooner said than done.

No-win situation

A situation where there is no satisfactory solution.

If the patient has surgery, it could result in many complications; if he doesn't have the surgery, the outcome is grave. It is a no-win situation.

Not all there

Not mentally adequate; crazy or silly.

Sometimes Cassie acts like she's not all there, causing her parents to worry about her well-being.

Not by a long shot

Not by any marked amount.

Did she complete the work assignment? No, not by a long shot!

Not for anything in the world

To refuse to do something regardless of the incentive.

When the doctor recommended surgery, the patient replied, "Not for anything in the world."

Not for love or money

To refuse to do something regardless of the incentive.

Lindsay would never consider moving away from her hometown – not for love or money.

Not hold water

To make no sense; to be illogical.

Your argument does not hold water.

Not one iota

Not even a tiny bit.

Hank told the doctor that not one iota of alcohol had crossed his lips in over 20 years.

Not up to scratch

Not adequate.

Sorry, your term paper is not up to scratch. You will have to redo it.

Nothing but skin and bones

Very thin.

The anorexic woman was nothing but skin and bones.

Null and void

Worthless.

I tore up the contract and the entire agreement became null and void.

Nutty as a fruitcake

Crazy.

Lynn does strange things that make people wonder if she is nutty as a fruitcake.

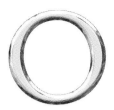

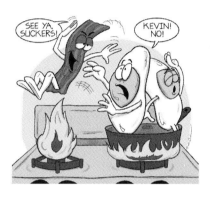

*Out of the frying pan
and into the fire*

Occur to (someone)

To have a thought or idea come into one's mind.

It occurred to Dr. Wells that he could try one last treatment option for Mrs. Janowski before he recommended surgery.

Odds and ends

Small, miscellaneous things.

The EMTs found lots of odds and ends in the back of the ambulance when they cleaned it out.

Of age

To be the legal age to do something.

June was of age, so she was able to have plastic surgery without parental consent.

Of all the nerve

Referring to a bold or shocking action or statement.

Brant walked out of the guest speaker's lecture. Of all the nerve!

Of all things

Referring to a surprising or unbelievable outcome.

Bridget went to the doctor because she had an upset stomach and was found to be six weeks pregnant, of all things.

Of benefit to

A positive occurrence for someone.

The new Women's Care Center will be of benefit to every woman from ages 18 to 80.

Of interest to

Of special importance to someone.

The new MRI will be of interest to surgeons who wish to rule out all other options before performing an invasive procedure.

Off and running

To get started up and functioning.

Dr. Peterson got his new practice off and running in just two months.

Off base

Incorrect.

The patient was off base when he said he could care for himself at home just as effectively as the nursing staff could care for him in the hospital.

Off chance

An unlikely possibility.

Dr. Lewis gave Rayleen the name of another obstetrician on the off chance that she went into premature labor while he was on vacation.

Off-color

Rude or vulgar.

The nurse reminded the patient his off-color jokes and remarks were inappropriate.

Off limits

Forbidden.

We cannot use the north wing of the hospital. It is being remodeled and is off limits for the next six months.

Off (one's) rocker

Crazy; silly.

Although Mrs. Harris often acted like she was off

her rocker, her doctor insisted that she wasn't se-
nile.

Off season

Not the busiest time of the year.

The emergency department does not have an off
season – every day is a busy day.

Off the air

Time during which a radio or TV program is not being
aired or shown.

Austin's favorite program went off the air at 11 p.m.

Off the beaten track

A remote or unknown area.

The little emergency clinic was off the beaten track,
so few people even knew it existed.

Off-the-cuff

Quick, spontaneous.

Emergency department physicians must be pre-
pared to make off-the-cuff diagnoses.

Off the record

An unofficial statement not intended for public knowledge.

Off the record, I disagree with Dr. Reilly's plan of
treatment.

Off the top of (one's) head

A quick response made without forethought.

Off the top of his head, Dr. Segal named five different therapies Margie could try in order to alleviate her back pain.

Off the wall

Unusual or silly.

Gavin thought that zero balancing sounded somewhat off the wall, but he was willing to try it in an attempt to relieve his recurring migraine headaches.

Off to a bad start

To start something (either a relationship or event) with negative factors or bad feelings.

The patient and the physician got off to a bad start.

Off to a running start

With a good, fast beginning.

The training sessions are off to a running start.

Old habits die hard

Activities or routines that one performs on a regular basis are difficult to discontinue because one has become accustomed to them.

Jerome knew he should stop smoking, but old habits die hard.

Old hand at (something)

Someone who is experienced at doing something.

After 20 years of experience, Bonnie is an old hand at transcription.

Old school

Ideas and methods that were once very useful and popular, but are no longer relevant.

Radical mastectomies are now old school; lumpectomies and partial resections are more modern options of treatment.

On a diet

An attempt to lose weight by restricting intake of certain foods.

To assist the patient in lowering her blood pressure, the doctor put her on a diet restricting fried and high-fat foods.

On a first name basis

To know someone very well.

The doctor and the patient were on a first name basis.

On a waiting list

Scheduled for an opportunity to do something.

The patient was placed on a waiting list for a kidney transplant.

On active duty

A military term referring to service during a combat situation.

All of the soldiers in the unit had to have physical exams before going on active duty.

On again, off again

Uncertain; indecisive.

The patient was on again, off again about scheduling surgery.

On call

Ready to serve when required.

The resident was on call when the patient went into cardiac arrest.

On easy street

In luxury.

Some people think if they win the lottery it will put them on easy street.

On edge

Anxious, nervous.

The patient's uncertain prognosis put him on edge.

On fire

Burning.

The patient told his physician that after eating a spicy meal, his stomach and chest felt like they were on fire.

On guard

To be cautious and mindful.

Although his injuries were mild and the altercation had been minor, the assault victim was still on guard when the paramedics arrived.

On medication

Currently taking a prescription drug to treat a medical condition.

Peggy's cardiologist put her on medication for high cholesterol and high blood pressure.

On occasion

Once in a while.

Generally, Ellen eats a very healthy and balanced diet, but on occasion she indulges in a piece of cake.

On (one's) feet again

Standing up; able to take care of oneself again.

After her car accident, Ruth had to move back in with her family, but only until she could recover enough to get on her feet again.

On (one's) honor

A promise made based on someone's integrity.

The patient was on his honor to take his medications properly.

On pins and needles

On edge; anxious.

The patient was on pins and needles waiting for the results of the test.

On probation

Under critical observation after committing a crime, causing trouble, or making a serious error.

After he misdiagnosed several patients, the hospital board of directors put Dr. Clark on probation.

On purpose

Deliberately.

Even though he suspected that Miss Dundlow had not hurt her child on purpose, the pediatrician still had to notify Social Services of the incident.

On second thought

To change one's mind about something after further consideration.

On second thought, let's not pursue this line of treatment further. We should try another protocol instead.

On (someone's) back

To continually nag or criticize someone.

Gerald felt like his doctor was always on his back about exercising.

On (someone's) case

To continually nag or criticize someone.

Mike hoped that the head resident wouldn't get on his case about being late for his shift at the hospital.

On (someone's) say-so

Based on a particular person's authority.

The nurse gave the patient additional pain medication on the doctor's say so.

On (someone's or something's) last legs

To be on the verge of giving up or dying.

The patient was so exhausted, she felt like she was on her last legs.

On standby

To be ready to do something on short notice.

The NICU team waited on standby as the triplets were delivered via cesarean section.

On target

Proceeding correctly; able to meet a deadline or adhere to a schedule.

Dr. Franz is confident that the therapy is on target and expects the patient to improve quickly.

On the alert

Watchful and attentive.

The doctor warned the patient to be on the alert for any change in the lump's size or shape.

On the ball

To be quick, alert, and efficient.

You have to be on the ball to work in the emergency department.

On the blink

Not functioning or working properly.

Dee's blood sugar monitor was on the blink, so she couldn't get an accurate reading of her levels.

On the contrary

The opposite of something.

Ann feared that the doctor would recommend prescription drugs to alleviate her arthritis pain, but she was surprised when, on the contrary, he advised complimentary and alternative medicine therapies.

On the double

Very fast.

Get over here, on the double!

On the eve of (something)

The night prior to a scheduled event.

On the eve of his surgery, Nigel was too nervous to sleep.

On the fritz

Not functioning or working properly.

The patient had to reschedule his x-ray appointment because the equipment was on the fritz.

On the go

Always busy.

The staff in the emergency department is always on the go.

On the heels of (something)

Soon after something.

The patient celebrated remission on the heels of completing radiation treatment.

On the hour

At each hour, on the hour mark.

Dr. Ling instructed the patient to take the medication every hour on the hour for three days.

On the job

Doing what one is expected to do.

The maternity ward nurse was on the job, getting ice for the moms-to-be, taking fetal heart readings, and performing various other tasks.

On the level

Honest, open, and fair.

Dr. Morris believes in being direct, so he always tries to be on the level with his patients regarding their diagnoses.

On the mend

Getting well; healing.

Trisha was on the mend from a sprained ankle, so

she had to miss her last two ballroom dancing classes.

On the money

To be exactly right about something.

Jack's self-diagnosis was on the money: His doctor confirmed that he had Lyme disease.

On the one hand; on the other hand

Presenting two opposing points of view.

On the one hand, the medication is extremely effective; on the other hand, there are serious side effects.

On the QT

Quietly; secretly.

Although visiting hours were over, the nurse gave the patient additional time with his family, on the QT.

On the right track

Heading in the right direction to achieve or discover something.

Following the prescribed program, the patient was on the right track for a full recovery.

On the rocks

A drink served with ice.

Susan ordered a margarita on the rocks with salt.

On the spot

In a difficult situation.

Leonard put his doctor on the spot when he asked for extra pain medication.

On the spur of the moment

Spontaneously or suddenly.

Darren sustained an injury to his ankle when, on the spur of the moment, he decided to jump into the pond, not realizing how shallow it was.

On the strength of

Based on the quality of something.

The patient was discharged on the strength of his promise to get plenty of rest, drink lots of fluids, and take his medications on time.

On the tip of (one's) tongue

On the verge of saying or remembering a specific fact.

The answer was on the tip of my tongue, but I just couldn't remember it.

On the up-and-up

Ethical, legal, and honest.

Dr. Klausen had a feeling that the patient was not on the up-and-up about her medical history.

On the verge of (something)

Just about to do something.

Tom was on the verge of quitting medical school, but his friend talked him out of it.

On the wagon

To abstain from something, usually alcohol or drugs.

Lilly had been on the wagon for five years since she'd undergone rehab for her drug addiction.

On the warpath

Angry and upset.

The doctor's condescending tone put the nurses on the warpath.

On the whole

Generally; overall.

On the whole, the MTs are doing a great job.

On thin ice

In a risky situation.

The patient was on thin ice for a while, but his condition is stable now.

Once and for all

Finally and irreversibly.

The store will close once and for all next week.

Once in a blue moon

Very rarely.

Dr. Davis only takes a day off from his private practice once in a blue moon.

Once-in-a-lifetime

A very rare opportunity or event.

Going on a trip around the world is a once-in-a-lifetime chance.

Once over

A quick examination.

I don't know how that doctor can be sure of his diagnosis since he only gave the patient a once over.

Once over lightly

A quick and careless examination.

The doctor gave the patient a once over lightly and then left the exam room.

Once upon a time

A long time ago; the phrase is usually used to begin a fairy tale.

Although she had gained 50 pounds during her pregnancy, Linda told Dr. Patterson that, once upon a time, she had a 24-inch waistline.

One and all

Everyone.

Eating fruits and vegetable is a healthy choice for one and all.

One and only

The only one; usually indicates that whatever is being referred to is unparalleled anywhere else.

The one and only free clinic in the area is located downtown.

One at a time

Individually.

The pharmacist counted out the capsules one at a time.

One by one

Individually.

The board interviewed 15 candidates, one by one, for the open resident position.

One in a million

Unique, unlike any other.

These days, physicians who make house calls are one in a million.

One jump ahead *or* One step ahead

Advanced in one's thinking or planning as compared to everyone else.

The ICU nurses always try to stay one jump ahead of their patients' needs.

One sandwich short of a picnic

Not very smart or logical.

When Dr. Travis recommended maggot therapy to

debride the wound, Hal wondered if he was one sandwich short of a picnic.

One too many

Too many; often refers to drinking too many alcoholic beverages.

The accident victim was slow to admit to the police that he had one too many at the bar before driving home.

One-track mind

To think entirely about a single subject.

Dr. Ramirez talks so much about sports it sometimes seems like he has a one-track mind, but he still treats his patients with the utmost care.

One way or another

Somehow.

Dallas was determined to get through medical school one way or another.

(One's) bark is worse than (one's) bite

One's threats or mannerisms are more frightening than their subsequent actions.

Dr. Kline's bedside manner can be rather brusque, but his bark is worse than his bite.

(One's) days are numbered

To face death or a dismissal.

Everyone realized that, unfortunately, the cancer patient's days were numbered.

(One's) heart goes out to (someone)

To feel compassion for someone.

My heart goes out to those who face life-challenging illnesses.

(One's) heart is in the right place

To have good intentions, even if the results are bad.

Although her heart was in the right place, the therapist couldn't convince the patient to stop using illegal drugs.

Open a can of worms

To uncover a set of problems.

In researching the cause of the accident, the inspector opened a can of worms.

Open-and-shut case

Something that is simple and straightforward.

The patient's symptoms were so obvious that diagnosing her was an open-and-shut case.

Open Pandora's box

To uncover many unsuspected problems.

The pharmaceutical company opened Pandora's box when they began researching the new heart drug and discovered numerous harmful side effects.

Out and about

Not at home; performing normal daily activities.

Once Ameet began feeling better, it wasn't long before he was out and about.

Out in left field

Offbeat; far from reality.

While we always welcome suggestions from our patients on how we can improve our care, I must admit that some of their ideas are really out in left field.

Out of character

Unlike one's usual behavior.

It was out of character for Leslie to be so short-tempered.

Out of control

Uncontrollable; wild.

The schizophrenic patient was out of control and had to be physically restrained.

Out of favor

No longer desirable or preferred.

The old cholesterol-lowering drug fell out of favor when the pharmaceutical company released a new one.

Out of hand

Unruly.

The crowd in the emergency department waiting room got out of hand.

Out of luck

To lack good fortune.

I got there too late and was out of luck finding a seat.

Out of nowhere

Suddenly; without warning.

According to the patient, an SUV appeared out of nowhere and struck the side of her car.

Out of the blue

Suddenly; without warning.

I was discussing the patient's menopause symptoms with her when, out of the blue, she told me she thought she might be pregnant.

Out of the clear blue sky

Suddenly; without warning.

One of the hikers reported that a bear appeared on the trail out of the clear blue sky, and the hikers knew they were in trouble.

Out of the frying pan and into the fire

From one bad situation to an even worse one.

Vince was out of the frying pan and into the fire when he crashed his truck right after he lost his job.

Out of the ordinary

Unusual.

Jill's symptoms were out of the ordinary for a normal sinus infection.

Out of the woods

Past a critical point.

The patient won't be out of the woods until his fever breaks.

Out on the town

To go out and have a good time, usually at a club or bar.

After passing their final exams, the class went out on the town to celebrate.

Out West

In the western part of the United States.

Do they still have cattle roundups out West?

Over and above (something)

More than something.

The cost of the plastic surgery was over and above what the doctor originally quoted to the patient.

Over and done with

Finished.

Denise hopes to make a full recovery once her treatment is over and done with.

Over the long haul

For a relatively long period of time.

The investment in the store should prove profitable over the long haul.

Over the short haul

For a relatively short period of time.

Although it's not a cure, acetaminophen should relieve your back pain over the short haul.

Over the top

To accomplish more than the expected goal.

The contributions from local high schools put the local charity drive over the top. They raised a record amount!

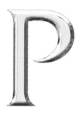

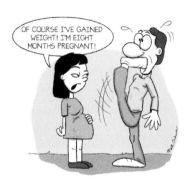

*Put your foot
in your mouth*

Pack a punch *or* Pack a wallop

To have a significant effect.

This antihistamine packs a wallop against allergy symptoms.

Packed in like sardines

Tightly squeezed into a space.

So many babies were born on the same day that they were packed in like sardines in the hospital nursery.

Pain in the neck *or* Pain in the rear *or* Pain in the butt

A bother.

Although taking medication every hour was a pain in the neck, Carol had to admit it made her feel better.

Paint the town red

To go out and celebrate.

Despite her doctor's orders, Kim went out and painted the town red. Subsequently, she suffered a setback.

Pale around the gills

To look sickly.

Andy had a few too many beers last night, so this morning he looks a little pale around the gills.

Par for the course

Typical or expected.

Nausea and hair loss are par for the course with chemotherapy.

Part and parcel

An essential part of something.

Rest, proper diet, and exercise are part and parcel of a good health regimen.

Part company

To leave someone.

Dr. Valdez wanted to start his own clinic, so he parted company with the group practice.

Pass away

To die.

The patient went into renal failure and passed away a short time later.

Pass out

To faint.

The patient went into shock and passed out in the waiting room.

Pass the buck

To deny responsibility for something and simultaneously place the blame on someone else.

The patient wasn't compliant with his doctor's orders, but he tried to pass the buck for his worsening condition by blaming his wife for not taking better care of him.

Pass the time

To occupy time by doing something.

While the patient was in surgery, the nurse encouraged his family to pass the time by reading or taking a walk.

Past (someone's or something's) prime

To have gone beyond the most useful, productive time.

The news program encouraged viewers to dispose of any medication past its prime.

Patch (someone or something) up

To repair something.

The doctor patched up the patient's wound with a few stitches and a bandage.

Path of least resistance

A course of action that requires minimal effort.

The patient was given several treatment options, and she chose the path of least resistance.

Pay an arm and a leg for (something)

To spend a great deal of money on something.

The patient complained that he had to pay an arm and a leg for his prescriptions.

Pay attention to (something or someone)

To focus on someone or something.

The nurse told Gerald to pay attention to his discharge orders and follow them carefully.

Pay (someone) a backhanded compliment

To offer someone a compliment that is really an insult.

Howard pays his wife a lot of backhanded compliments, but he does it in such a good-natured way that she doesn't take too much offense.

Pay (someone) a visit

To go to see someone.

After her discharge, the patient's family came to her house to pay her a visit.

Pay the piper

To face the consequences of one's own actions.

The patient was not compliant with the doctor's orders and had to pay the piper when he was readmitted to the hospital.

Pay through the nose

To spend a great deal of money on something.

The insurance company had to pay through the nose to cover the patient's claim.

Penny-wise and pound-foolish

To place more emphasis on the insignificant details of a situation than the overall outcome.

Brenda thought it was a good idea to save money by buying a generic cough syrup, but she realized she'd been penny-wise and pound-foolish when it didn't work and she was up all night coughing.

Pep up (someone)

To energize someone.

The afternoon break helped to pep up the staff.

Perk (someone) up

To energize or cheer up someone.

The good news from the lab seemed to perk the patient up immediately.

Peter out

To become tired; to dwindle away slowly.

The patient complained that he petered out after walking just a short distance.

Pick a quarrel *or* Pick a fight

To attempt to start an argument.

Lucia was accused of being argumentative and trying to pick a quarrel with the nursing staff.

Pick at (someone)

To verbally reprimand someone on an ongoing basis.

Janie picked at her husband to take better care of himself until he finally stopped smoking and started exercising.

Pick (someone's) brain

To extract information from someone.

The psychologist picked Dave's brain to try to determine why he continued his self-destructive behavior.

Pick (something or someone) to pieces

To severely criticize something or someone.

Louis was unhappy with his accommodations and picked everything to pieces until the nurse arranged to transfer him to another room.

Pick up the check *or* Pick up the tab

To pay for something.

Jaime picked up the check for the lunch.

Piece of cake

An easy or simple task.

Andrea was anxious to get out of bed, so getting her ambulatory again was a piece of cake for the physical therapist.

Pinch-hit

To fill in for someone.

Dr. Green was pinch-hitting for Dr. Rawlings yesterday.

Pipe down

To become quiet.

The nurse came to the room to ask the patient to pipe down, as he was disturbing the other patients on the floor.

Pit (someone) against (someone else)

To create a situation that causes two individuals to become adversaries.

The doctor feared that his controversial recommendation would pit Mr. Sims against the rest of his family.

Plain and simple

Easy; without complication.

The nurse kept the instructions plain and simple.

Play both ends against the middle

To manipulate people or situations.

Miguel was quite good at playing both ends against the middle in order to get his way.

Play-by-play description

To give a detailed account of something.

Haley gave a play-by-play description of the accident to the ED doctor.

Play cat and mouse

To treat someone cruelly then kindly; to repeatedly draw someone close then push him or her away.

The patient played cat and mouse with the hospital staff, rather than being forthright and honest with them.

Play devil's advocate

To create an argument to stimulate thought and ideas.

At the patient treatment review board, the doctors took turns playing devil's advocate to make sure they considered all the available options and outcomes.

Play hardball

To be aggressive and unwavering in a situation.

The insurance company played hardball with the patient's claim, refusing to pay it.

Play havoc

To confuse or disrupt.

Kenny misbehaved at school again, playing havoc with the teacher.

Play hooky

To be intentionally absent from a scheduled event or appointment.

Rather than attend the lecture, Oscar and Misty played hooky and went to the beach instead.

Play into (someone's) hands

To manipulate someone into becoming part of a scheme without their knowledge.

May played right into Tina's hands and ended up doing the majority of the work on the project without even realizing it.

Play it cool

To remain calm.

Jesse played it cool when he was questioned, so the nurse had no idea he'd stolen the pain medication.

Play it safe

To take all precautions.

Even though her fever has broken, we should play it safe and take Iris in for a checkup.

Play possum

To pretend to be inactive or asleep.

Alicia did not want to get up and do her homework, so she played possum when her mother came in to check on her.

Play second fiddle

To be less important or have less status than someone else.

Frank played second fiddle to Mark, since Mark had more experience.

Play (someone) against (someone else)

To create a situation that causes two individuals to become adversaries.

Carrie Ann was good at playing her mother against her father to get her way.

Play with fire

To take a substantial risk.

Dr. Goodings warned the patient that if he did not take the medications properly, he'd be playing with fire and could become seriously ill.

Plow into (something or someone)

To hit something at a high rate of speed.

The accident victim remembers plowing into the bus, but then she lost consciousness and does not know what happened after that.

Plug (something) up

To fill a gap; to stop the flow of a liquid.

The EMT used gauze to plug up the open chest wound.

Plum crazy

Completely out of one's mind.

Mr. Braud went plum crazy when he learned about his daughter's illness.

Point of no return

A critical juncture in which the only option is to proceed.

The patient was at the point of no return in his therapy.

Pour (one's) heart out

To confess everything to someone.

The patient poured her heart out to her psychologist.

Powers that be

The people in control of a situation; those in positions of authority.

It is up to the powers that be at the insurance company as to whether Ms. Sharpe will be transferred or not.

Presence of mind

The ability to act sensibly.

In the face of a possible crisis, the patient's wife had the presence of mind to call 911.

Pressed for time

To be in a rush.

The doctor wanted to talk with Salama and her family but was pressed for time, so he asked if he could reschedule their appointment for the next day.

Prevail upon (someone)

To convince or persuade someone.

Can I prevail upon you to assist me?

Psyche (someone) out

To cause someone to worry about something unnecessarily.

With all his talk about the pain and agony that she would experience, Brandi's brother psyched her out about having her wisdom teeth removed.

Psyche (someone) up (for something)

To mentally prepare for something.

The patient tried to psyche himself up for the surgery, but was still a little scared.

Pull (one's) own weight

To do one's share.

Everyone is going to need to pull his or her own weight for the project to succeed.

Pull (oneself) up by the bootstraps

To get ahead unaided, through one's own perseverance and diligence.

Frieda is a perfect example of how someone can start life with nothing and pull themselves up by the bootstraps to achieve success.

Pull out all the stops

To use all one's energy and resources.

The doctor pulled out all the stops to save the little girl.

Pull some strings

To use one's influence.

The doctor had to pull some strings to get Mr. Valentino admitted to a private room.

Pull (someone or something) down

To adversely affect someone.

Don't let Gene's bad mood pull you down, too.

Pull through

To survive a situation.

The operation was successful, and the patient should pull through with no complications.

Push the envelope

To press on to surpass the expected limitation.

Even though Jason had been running 10 miles a day, he added another 5 miles, which was really pushing the envelope.

Put all (one's) eggs in one basket

To place confidence in only one thing; to rely on only one source.

Rather than making the lifestyle changes his doctor recommended, Ed put all his eggs in one basket, counting on the cholesterol medication to cure his heart disease.

Put ideas into (someone's) head

To persuade someone to do or think something that they otherwise would not.

Be careful what you say to him; you might put ideas in his head.

Put off by (someone or something)

To be offended by someone or something.

The patient was put off by the attendant's behavior.

Put on airs

To behave as if you are superior to everyone else; to act conceited.

To hide her insecurity, Amy puts on airs around people that she does not know and often ends up alienating them with her snooty behavior.

Put on an act

To pretend.

Be yourself! Putting on an act will get you nowhere.

Put (one's) foot in (one's) mouth

To say something inappropriate, hurtful, or insulting; to make a silly verbal blunder.

Tim criticized the way the meeting was run before he realized that the president was standing behind him. He really put his foot in his mouth.

Put (one's) nose to the grindstone

To work diligently.

Transcription takes a great deal of concentration, so you really have to put your nose to the grindstone.

Put (one's) two cents in

To offer one's opinion.

Paul interrupted the doctor to put his two cents in about which treatment he preferred.

Put (someone or something) through the wringer

To put someone or something through the most difficult of situations.

Margo really put Marian through the wringer during the interview, asking her one difficult question after another.

Put (someone or something) to the test

To determine the abilities and potential of someone or something.

The doctor decided to put the new arthritis drug to the test by prescribing it to some of his patients.

Put (something) on the back burner

To make something less of a priority.

We are not sure how to proceed with this project, so for now we will put it on the back burner.

Put (something) plainly

To make something simple; to say something in a way that is easy to understand.

Carl experienced a myocardial infarction, or, to put it plainly, a heart attack.

Put (something) through the paces

To demonstrate the extent of someone's or something's capabilities.

The physical therapist put the patient through the paces to see how much additional therapy she would need before she could be discharged from the hospital.

Put the cart before the horse

To put things in the wrong order; to think too far into the future without considering the present circumstances.

Dr. Carroll put the cart before the horse when he began planning the expansion of the neurology wing before receiving confirmation the funds would be approved.

Put the kibosh on (something)

To put an end to something.

Since this therapy is not working, I will put the kibosh on it and start a new regimen Monday.

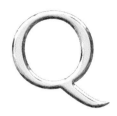

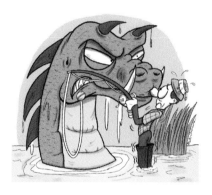

Quake in one's boots

Quake in (one's) boots

To be afraid.

Quinn was quaking in her boots waiting for her test results to come back.

Quick as a flash

Very fast.

The doctor moved quick as a flash to get the patient out of the ambulance.

Quick as greased lightening

With great speed.

When the nurse sounded a Code Blue in the pa-

tient's room, the rest of the team arrived quick as greased lightening.

Quick on the trigger

To give a speedy response.

When the orderly asked what Franklin was doing in a restricted area of the hospital, he was quick on the trigger with an answer.

Quick on the uptake

To promptly process and comprehend information.

Emergency department personnel must be quick on the uptake in order to treat patients efficiently and effectively.

Quiet as a mouse

Almost silent.

The NICU nurse moved from incubator to incubator as quiet as a mouse so that she wouldn't wake the sleeping infants.

Quite a bit

A lot of something.

Cindy experienced quite a bit more postsurgical pain than she expected.

Quite a few

Many.

The patient experienced quite a few unanticipated side effects while on the anticonvulsant drug.

Quite a lot

Much.

The nurse had to remove quite a lot of debris from the accident victim's wounds.

Quote a price

To provide an estimate of the cost of an item or service before it is purchased.

Prior to admission, Ms. Coppinger asked the surgery center to quote a price on the procedure.

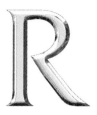

R

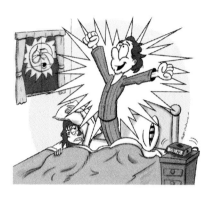

Rise and shine

Race against time

To move quickly.

The organ transplant team raced against time to replace the patient's failing kidney with the one his brother donated to him.

Rack (one's) brain

To try very hard to think of something.

The toddler's parents racked their brains to think of what the child might have ingested to make him so sick.

Racked with pain

Suffering extreme discomfort.

When the patient was admitted to the emergency department he was racked with pain, so the attending physician gave him a shot of morphine.

Rain cats and dogs

A heavy downpour of rain.

The ambulance had trouble getting to the hospital quickly because it was raining cats and dogs.

Rain on (someone's) parade

To ruin someone's plans or to diminish their enthusiasm or happiness.

The therapist hated to rain on Naomi's parade, but he told her that she hadn't made adequate progress.

Rain or shine

No matter what; regardless of the weather conditions.

The benefit auction for the cancer ward was scheduled to take place at the pier the following Saturday, rain or shine.

Raise a stink

To create a disturbance.

Violet threatened to raise a stink about the increased prescription drug co-pays outlined in her insurance plan.

Raise an objection

To bring up a concern or complaint about something or someone.

The patient raised an objection to having another physician consult on his case.

Raise Cain *or* Raise hell

To create a disturbance.

When Armando found out the doctor was running late, he raised Cain in the clinic reception area.

Raise eyebrows

To cause concern, surprise, or dismay.

Terrence's erratic behavior raised eyebrows among the emergency department staff, so they called in someone from the psych ward to evaluate his mental state.

Raise havoc

To disrupt something or create difficulty.

When he didn't take his antipsychotic medication, Perry's behavior raised havoc in the classroom and other social settings.

Raise (one's) voice

To speak very loudly.

The patient raised his voice when he became upset during his therapy session.

Raise the dickens

To behave in an extreme manner.

Physicians will often raise the dickens with the nursing staff if they provide incompetent patient care.

Rake (someone) over the coals

To severely scold someone.

The HMO claims representative raked Becky over the coals for not submitting her insurance premium payment on time.

Rally around (something or someone)

To come together to provide support to someone or something.

The campaign supporters rallied around the presidential candidate because of his stance on Medicare reform.

Ram (something) down (someone's) throat

To force something on someone.

The nutritionist believed so strongly in high-protein, low-carbohydrate diets that she tried to ram them down all her client's throats.

Ramble on

To talk aimlessly.

Mr. Griffin rambled on for half an hour about the minute details of his medical history.

Rant and rave

To speak in a very agitated, angry manner.

The patient began to rant and rave uncontrollably and had to be sedated.

Rap with (someone)

To talk with someone.

The support group members liked to rap with one another about their experiences.

Rat on (someone) *or* Rat (someone) out

To reveal someone's wrongdoing to an authoritative figure.

Jared's wife ratted on him to his urologist about his failure to take his medication for benign prostatic hypertrophy.

Rattle off (something)

To recite something very quickly.

The patient rattled off his list of complaints and problems faster than the nurse could write them down.

Reach a compromise

To arrive at a solution or conclusion that both sides of an opposing issue find satisfactory.

After many hours of discussion, the team of doctors reached a compromise on how to proceed with Mr. Cole's treatment.

Reach an agreement

To arrive at a decision that both sides of an opposing issue find satisfactory.

The committee didn't reach an agreement on the new HIPAA policies until after midnight.

Reach an impasse

To progress to a point where an obstacle or disagreement prevents further discussion on an issue.

Vaughn and his doctor reached an impasse when Vaughn refused further treatment.

Reach first base

To accomplish the first goal needed to continue further.

The therapist worked hard to gain the patient's trust, and felt that they had reached first base by the end of the session.

Reach for the sky

To aspire to attain something that seems practically impossible.

The physical therapist encouraged Shirley to reach for the sky in her pursuit to regain the use of her legs.

Read between the lines

To interpret something from contextual clues.

The doctor responded to Walter's questions about his prognosis with vague answers, but Walter could read between the lines.

Read into (something)

To overanalyze something in an attempt to determine an underlying meaning.

Even though the doctor was very open and reassuring with her, Sue kept trying to read something else into what he was saying.

Read (someone) like an open book

To easily interpret someone's thoughts or feelings based on their body language and physical reactions.

After 20 years as his primary care physician, Dr. Leonard could read Tim like an open book.

Read (someone) (one's) rights

To provide the Miranda Rights to someone being arrested.

When the police captured the thief, they read him his rights as they put the handcuffs on him.

Read (someone) the riot act

To severely reprimand someone.

Dr. Yates read the patient the riot act when he found out he wasn't taking his medications properly.

Read (something) over

To review a written document.

Dr. Diaz gave the case report to Dr. Czerniak so he could read it over before seeing the patient for a second opinion.

Read the handwriting on the wall *or* Read the writing on the wall

To predict the outcome of something.

Although he had hoped to beat his prostate cancer, Larry could read the handwriting on the wall.

Read up on (something)

To gain knowledge about something through research.

The doctor was unfamiliar with Andy's condition, so he wanted to read up on it before proceeding with the exam.

Ready and willing *or* Ready, willing, and able

Eager and capable of doing something.

The patient was ready, willing, and able to begin physical therapy.

Real thing

Genuine.

Nicole found it difficult to follow her nutritionist's recommendation to switch from ice cream to frozen yogurt. She preferred the real thing.

Reality of the situation

The truth.

Frank believes that he is almost finished with his therapy, but the reality of the situation is that he still hasn't made adequate progress.

Rear (its) ugly head

For something unpleasant to surface.

When the Centers for Disease Control released its annual mortality report, the dismal pancreatic cancer survival rate reared its ugly head.

Reckon with (something or someone)

To deal with something or someone.

The doctor had a great deal of difficulty reckoning with the patient's reaction to his diagnosis.

Reconcile (oneself) to (something)

To accept a situation.

The patient must reconcile herself to the gravity of her illness and comply with the recommended course of treatment.

Red-carpet treatment

Special, often to the point of luxurious, treatment.

Luke got the red-carpet treatment in the hospital, with a private room and personalized meals.

Red herring

Information intended to divert attention away from the truth.

The psychologist concluded that Harriet's frequent complaints about her family members were simply a red herring so she could avoid taking responsibility for her own inability to effectively communicate with others.

Red in the face

Embarrassed.

Jane turned red in the face when she realized she had been overheard.

Red tape

A set of complicated regulations or procedures that delay the final outcome of a situation.

Filing an insurance claim involves a lot of red tape.

Reduced to

To be brought down to a humbled state.

The patient was reduced to tears when the doctor diagnosed her with multiple sclerosis.

Regain (one's) composure

To become calm following a period of agitation.

The patient found it difficult to regain her composure after arguing with her mother.

Regardless of

Despite something.

Regardless of the cost or the amount of time involved, the patient wanted to take advantage of every modality available to treat his illness.

Regular as clockwork

Absolutely dependable.

The patient took her medication as regular as clockwork: She never missed a dose.

Reminiscent of (something)

To remind someone of someone or something else.

The new drug ads make outrageous claims that are reminiscent of the techniques used years ago by snake-oil salesmen.

Reputed to be

Considered by many to have certain qualities or characteristics.

Dr. Wu is reputed to be the best hand surgeon in the United States.

Resign (oneself) to (something)

To accept reluctantly.

The patient resigned herself to a long course of physical therapy.

Rest assured

To be certain about something.

HIPAA regulations allow patients to rest assured that their privacy will be protected.

Rest on (one's) laurels

To enjoy the success one has attained without progressing further.

John rested on his laurels rather than making additional efforts to prove he was worthy of the head resident position.

Result in (something)

To cause something to happen.

Extended use of some drugs may result in serious side effects and other complications.

Return the favor

To do something good for someone who has done something good for you.

Mark thanked the other intern for switching shifts with him and promised to return the favor.

Rev (something) up

To incite action.

Dr. Mills told Caitlin that exercise would help rev up her metabolism.

Rich in (something)

To have a lot of something.

Oranges are rich in vitamin C.

Ride on (someone's) coattails

To make your good fortune by taking advantage of someone else's success.

When Dr. Zechman made a name for himself with his ground-breaking research, his assistant was more than willing to ride his coattails to success.

Ride roughshod over (someone or something)

To treat someone or something with scorn or lack of respect.

The doctors ride roughshod over the residents and interns.

Ride (something) out

To endure something that is unpleasant.

The treatment was physically grueling, but the patient rode it out.

Ride the gravy train

To live in luxury.

Paolo chose to specialize in plastic surgery, hoping that the high salary would soon have him riding the gravy train.

Riding for a fall

Risking failure.

Lowell has been warned about his cholesterol count, so he's riding for a fall by eating fried foods.

Right as rain

Correct.

Nadia said the computers for the new MTs would be delivered on Friday and she was as right as rain.

Right down (someone's) alley

Perfectly suited to someone's talents or preferences.

Brooke loves children, so becoming a pediatrician seems to be right down her alley.

Right off the bat

Immediately.

The doctor knew what was wrong with Rico right off the bat.

Right on time

According to schedule.

The patient arrived for her appointment right on time, but was kept waiting for over an hour.

Right up (someone's) alley

Perfectly suited to someone's talents or preferences.

Carrie enjoys typing, so medical transcription is right up her alley.

Ring true

To sound familiar or applicable to someone or something.

The doctor's description of fibromyalgia rang true with Alicia's symptoms.

Ripe old age

Very old age.

The patient lived to the ripe old age of 104.

Ripple of excitement

Quiet enthusiasm.

The announcement of the new hyperbaric chamber caused a ripple of excitement at the staff meeting.

Rise and shine

To wake up and get out of bed.

Leann still felt tired, but she knew she had to rise and shine if she wanted to make it to her shift on time.

Rise to the occasion *or* Rise to the challenge

To meet a challenge.

The research team rose to the occasion and determined the microorganism responsible for the outbreak.

Risk (one's) neck

To accept the possibility of danger or bodily harm in order to accomplish something.

Since his allergic reaction wasn't too severe, Steve just drove to the hospital slowly rather than risking his neck by speeding.

Road hog

A inconsiderate driver.

That road hog is making it impossible for the ambulance to get through.

Rob Peter to pay Paul

To take from one to give to another.

Sometimes in the emergency department supplies are borrowed from another area. It's like robbing Peter to pay Paul.

Rock the boat

To disturb a situation that is otherwise stable.

Dr. Singleton preferred not to rock the boat by introducing a new drug into the patient's current regimen.

Roll over in (one's) grave

To do something so shocking that it would cause even a deceased person to react.

If Hannah's grandmother knew that her grand-daughter had breast augmentation surgery, she would roll over in her grave.

Roll up (one's) sleeves

To prepare to do work.

Mark wanted to assist in the appendectomy, so he rolled up his sleeves and started prepping for surgery.

Rolling stone gathers no moss

A proverb that states that constant movement prevents substantial material, physical, or personal gain.

The homeless man was encouraged to stay put long enough to get tretment, but he preferred to move on. A rolling stone gathers no moss.

Rome wasn't built in a day

A proverb that states that anything that is vital or important takes time to develop.

Bailey got discouraged with her slow recovery pro-

gress, but her therapist reminded her that Rome wasn't built in a day.

Rotten to the core

Very bad or immoral.

Dr. Logan's billing procedures were rotten to the core and caused the authorities to revoke his medical license.

Rough idea

A general overview or a loose explanation.

The doctor gave the patient a rough idea as to how he wanted to proceed with treatment.

Rough it

To do without luxuries or amenities.

When Tammy went into labor in the middle of a blizzard, she and her husband had to rough it and deliver their baby at home.

Rough (someone) up

To physically harm someone.

The gas station attendant called 911 after being roughed up by armed robbers.

Royal treatment

Special and extravagant gestures.

When Mr. Finlay expressed his dismay at having to share a hospital room with another patient, the nurse told him not to expect royal treatment.

Rub elbows with (someone)

To be close to someone in a given situation.

Dr. Gordon hoped to be awarded a research grant, so he sought out every opportunity to rub elbows with members of the decision-making committee.

Rub salt in a wound

To purposely make someone feel worse than they already do.

Nancy found her weight gain very discouraging, but Len rubbed salt in the wound by telling her that she should have followed her diet more carefully.

Rub (someone) the wrong way

To offend or irritate someone.

For some reason, Nurse Robinson always rubs patients the wrong way.

Rub (someone's) nose in (something)

To remind someone of something that they have done wrong.

Shawna reminded Gino she was making more progress than he was, and he asked her not to rub his nose in it.

Ruffle (one's) feathers

To annoy or offend someone.

The doctor did not have a very good bedside manner: He tended to ruffle his patients' feathers.

Rule of thumb

A general, unofficial guideline.

As a rule of thumb, most patients should expect several months of therapy following knee replacement surgery.

Run a fever

To have an elevated body temperature.

Mrs. Neiman reported that her baby had been running a fever all night.

Run a tight ship

To operate something in a disciplined, strict manner.

The head nurse of the maternity ward runs a tight ship to prevent any chaos from disturbing the babies and mothers.

Run around like a chicken with its head cut off

To be disorganized and frantic.

When her husband had a heart attack, Millicent panicked and ran around like a chicken with its head cut off.

Run in the family

To occur in many of one's relatives.

Heart disease runs in the patient's family.

Run like clockwork

To proceed smoothly.

The grand opening of the new women's clinic ran like clockwork.

Run-of-the-mill

Common.

Madison didn't have a specific complaint, she just went to her doctor for a run-of-the-mill physical exam.

Run off at the mouth

To talk excessively.

Many of the psychologist's patients tend to run off at the mouth during their sessions, and she encourages them to express all of their feelings.

Run out of patience

To become frustrated.

The doctor ran out of patience with his assistant when she took too long to prepare the inoculation.

Run (someone) ragged

To keep someone very busy.

Gil's physical therapist runs him ragged during his weekly sessions.

Run (something) by (someone)

To seek someone's opinion about an idea, thought, or plan.

Before she gave the patient a pain reliever, the nurse ran it by the attending physician.

Run the gambit

To exhaust all options.

The patient was willing to try a new medication, but the doctor explained they had run the gambit of what was available.

Run the risk

Take a chance.

We could put the patient on the new drug, but we run the risk of terrible side effects.

Rustle (something) up

To find or create something using limited resources.

Dr. Zandier rustled up some free samples of cough medication for Mrs. Williams.

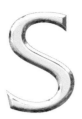

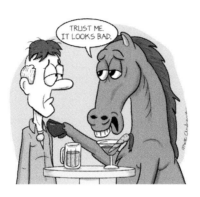

*Straight from
the horse's mouth*

Sack out

To fall asleep.

Mr. Hall reports that he is so tired after a day at work that he sacks out at about 8 p.m. every night.

Sacred cow

Something regarded with a great deal of respect and reverence.

The statin drug had worked so well for his patients that Dr. Bryant seemed to regard it as a sacred cow.

Sadder but wiser

Unhappy, but better educated about something or someone.

Maureen's facelift didn't turn out the way she expected, and now she's sadder but wiser about plastic surgery.

Saddle (someone) with (something)

To burden someone with something.

Bernie did not want to saddle the doctor with all his problems.

Safe and sound

Secure and healthy.

The baby arrived safe and sound!

Safety in numbers

To be more secure in a large group.

The ladies walked together in a group, knowing that there was safety in numbers.

Sail right through (something)

To complete something easily.

Payton sailed right through his medical licensing exams.

Salt of the earth

Someone who is very ethical and practical and prefers a simple way of life.

Dr. Martinez is the salt of the earth and would fit in

better in a rural country clinic than he does in the
busy city hospital.

Same here

To verbally agree with someone.

After one of the people at the Narcotics Anonymous
meeting admitted to relapsing, another person came
forward and said, "Same here."

Same old story

To relate something that has happened over and over
again.

Every time he sees his doctor, Mr. Reed relates the
same old story about pain in his lower joints.

Save face

To preserve one's dignity or good standing.

The pharmaceutical company spent millions of dol-
lars on a new advertising campaign in order to save
face after a scandal broke out regarding one of its
products.

Save (one's) breath

To refrain from saying something or giving advice because anything that is said will not be heeded.

Dr. Edison knew he wouldn't convince Barbara to
quit smoking, so he saved his breath.

Save (something) for a rainy day

To reserve something for a special purpose or time of
need.

Joanie wanted to save her movie passes for a rainy day.

Save the day

To rescue someone or correct a situation.

Just when the surgical team thought the patient wouldn't survive, Dr. James saved the day with his quick thinking.

Saved by the bell

To be rescued from a difficult or undesirable situation.

Forrest was saved by the bell when his medication took effect just before his condition deteriorated permanently.

Saving grace

A genuinely positive characteristic.

Although this procedure is complicated and time consuming, its saving grace is that it is inexpensive.

Say a mouthful

To say something of significance; to imply something much larger than what has actually been said.

When Haley said the MTs were busy, she said a mouthful.

Say (something) in a roundabout way

To imply or hint at something.

When speaking to a patient, it is better to be direct rather than saying something in a roundabout way.

Say the word

To give a verbal signal for action.

The nurse told Bob to just say the word if he needed more pain medication.

Say uncle

To give in or surrender.

Dr. Coleman forced the patient to say uncle by withholding pain medication until she promised to comply fully with his orders.

Scare (someone) out of (one's) wits

To become extremely frightened.

When Wesley stopped breathing, it scared his wife out of her wits.

Scare the living daylights out of (someone) *or* Scare the devil out of (someone) *or* Scare the dickens out of (someone)

To terrify someone.

When the DOA patient opened his eyes, it scared the living daylights out of the emergency room physician.

Scrape the bottom of the barrel

To be forced to select from the poorest options.

The inner city clinic was so understaffed that its administrators had no choice but to scrape the bottom of the barrel when hiring nurses.

Scratch the surface

To gain only limited knowledge about or experience with something.

Researchers have only scratched the surface of the healing potential of herbs.

Scream bloody murder

To yell and shriek loudly; to make a scene.

The young child was afraid to receive the injection, and he screamed bloody murder when the nurse approached him with the syringe.

Scrimp and save

To sacrifice and gather funds over time in order to attain something.

The Hernandez family scrimped and saved to pay for their daughter's bone marrow transplant.

Seamy side of life

The unpleasant, immoral aspects of the world.

When he was hooked on heroin, Leo saw the seamy side of life.

Second nature to (someone)

To have a special talent for something.

Dr. Kelly is a very talented cardiac surgeon, and coronary bypass surgeries are like second nature to him.

See double

To see two of everything.

During the accident, the patient suffered damage to part of his brain, causing him to see double.

See eye to eye

To agree.

Although mainstream doctors and complementary medicine doctors disagree on many points, they do see eye to eye on the importance of a healthy diet and exercise.

See no objection to (something or someone)

To be unable to find a reason why something should not occur.

The doctor could see no objection to the patient getting out of bed.

See (one's) way clear to (do something)

To find it possible to do something.

Jackson saw his way clear to leave work early in order to get to his therapy session on time.

See red

To be very angry.

Brandy saw red when the nurse told her she wouldn't be discharged that day.

See (something) through

To finish something.

Medical residency is extremely demanding, but those who see it through feel their efforts were well worth it.

See stars

To see flashes of lights.

The patient complained of seeing stars after being hit on the head.

See the handwriting on the wall *or* See the writing on the wall

To know for certain that something is going to happen.

After the last round of chemotherapy failed to put Leslie's cancer into remission, everyone could see the handwriting on the wall and knew that she wouldn't survive much longer.

See the light

To come to a realization; to understand another's way of thinking.

After Dr. Parker explained the procedure further, the patient finally saw the light and agreed to go through with it.

See which way the wind blows

To determine what is likely to happen in a particular situation.

We will assess all the therapeutic options and see which way the wind is blowing in terms of treating the patient's neuropathy.

Seen better days

Worn out; not in peak condition.

The current dictation system has seen better days. It is time to upgrade to newer technology.

Seize the bull by the horns

To confront something and deal with it.

Rather than drawing out his decision, Robert seized the bull by the horns and chose to have exploratory surgery right away.

Sell like hotcakes

To sell very quickly.

As soon as Claritin became available without a prescription, it started selling like hotcakes.

Sell (someone) on (something)

To convince someone of the benefits of something.

The pharmaceutical company had to sell the FDA on the safety and effectiveness of its new drug in order to gain approval.

Send (someone) packing

To dismiss or fire someone.

Dr. Benitez sent his assistant packing when she lost a patient's records for the third time in one month.

Separate but equal

Different but of the same status.

Miss Barnes felt that acupuncture was a separate but equal way of treating her persistent migraines.

Separate the men from the boys

To determine which members of a group are most worthy.

Residents are put through long shifts in order to separate the men from the boys and see which ones can handle the tedious schedules required of physicians.

Set a precedent

To establish a new standard.

Nasir's outstanding success with the recently-developed protocol set a precedent for fibromyalgia treatment.

Set great store in (someone or something)

To have absolute confidence in someone or something.

The patient set great store in his doctor's abilities.

Set in (one's) ways

To be resistant to change.

The doctor had a hard time getting Isaac to comply with his order to begin an exercise program because he was so set in his ways.

Set (one's) sights on (something)

To establish something as a goal.

The patient set his sights on completing therapy by October.

Set (someone) back

To cost someone a certain amount of money.

The blood pressure medication set Paul back $65 a month.

Set (someone or something) straight

To correct a misunderstanding or mistake.

Carol didn't understand her HMO's deductible procedures, but the insurance company customer service representative set her straight.

Set (something) back

To delay something.

Missing just two physical therapy sessions set Uri's progress back substantially.

Set up shop

To start a business.

Dr. Munz is going to set up shop in the north section of town.

Settle down

To become calm.

Although he was having a lot of fun with his visitors, Dwayne's nurse told him to settle down so as not to disturb the other patients on the floor.

Settle for (something)

To accept a less-than-desirable offer.

Erma preferred the brand name drug, but she told the pharmacist she would settle for the generic version.

Shake hands on (something)

A verbal agreement between two people, culminated in a handshake.

Dr. Carlito and Stewart agreed to meet the following week to discuss further treatment options and shook hands on it.

Shake in (one's) boots

To be afraid.

Quincy was shaking in his boots wondering if his wife would survive her triple bypass surgery.

Shake (someone) up

To become upset or disoriented.

The first time she had a panic attack, it really shook Cheryl up because she thought she was having a heart attack.

Shape up

To improve one's behavior or physical or mental condition.

Josie started an aerobic and weight-training regimen to shape up for the marathon.

Shape up or ship out

To choose to improve one's behavior or leave.

The patient continued to treat the nurse rudely so she told him to shape up or ship out.

Sharp as a knife *or* Sharp as a razor *or* Sharp as a tack

Mentally acute.

Dr. Brandt is as sharp as a razor and is often able to diagnose his patients after just a few minutes.

Shed light on (something)

To clarify something.

Tina learned a great deal about herself during her counseling sessions because her therapist shed light on the subconscious reasons for her behavior.

Shell out

To pay a certain amount of money for something.

Jed had to shell out $500 to meet his insurance company's deductible.

Shirk (one's) duties

To ignore an assigned task or job.

The resident always shirks his duties at the end of each shift and does an inadequate job of completing his paperwork.

Shoot the breeze

To chat with someone in a casual manner.

Dr. Ahmed wished he had more time to shoot the

breeze with his patients, but his busy schedule didn't permit it.

Short and sweet *or* Short, sweet, and to the point
Brief.

The doctor kept his dictation short and sweet.

Short of (something)
To not have enough of something.

The hospital was short of Demerol, so Dr. Sheriton had to give the patient a different pain medication.

Shot in the dark
A guess.

The doctor had never encountered symptoms like Grant's, so he took a shot in the dark when ordering his lab tests.

Shoulder to shoulder
Side by side; in close proximity.

The National Academy of Science conference was so crowded that attendees were shoulder to shoulder during some of the presentations.

Show (one's) true colors
To reveal one's actual personality or characteristics.

When she doesn't take her mood-stabilizing medication, Charlotte reveals her true colors.

Show (someone) the ropes

To assist someone in learning an established set of procedures.

The emergency department was so busy that no one had time to show the new interns the ropes.

Shy away from (something)

To avoid or retreat from something.

Although she is slowly overcoming her agoraphobia, Gena still shies away from crowds.

Sick and tired

To be frustrated and irritated with something or someone.

The patient was sick and tired of trying new medications.

Side with (someone)

To support someone's actions or point of view.

Mr. Coppock's wife sided with his decision to discontinue his radiation treatments.

Sight for sore eyes

A welcome arrival.

After three months of being fed intravenously, Darren considered solid food a sight for sore eyes.

Simmer down

To calm down after being agitated or upset.

The nurse attempted to get the patient to simmer down before the doctor arrived.

Sing (someone's or something's) praises

To commend someone or something.

Many people who have had gastric bypass surgery sing its praises.

Sink in

To absorb knowledge.

It took several days for it to sink in to Andrea that she was pregnant.

Sink (one's) teeth into (something)

To delve into a project or other activity; *also*, to take a bite of food.

Mark had prepared well for the project and was ready to sink his teeth into it.

After eliminating red meat from his diet for six months, Howard looked forward to sinking his teeth into a juicy steak.

Sink or swim

Something or someone will either fail miserably or be a great success.

The researchers initiated a clinical trial on the new drug to determine whether it would sink or swim.

Sit in for (someone)

To take someone's place.

Dr. Aldy can't be at the hospital board meeting, so his assistant will sit in for him.

Sit (something) out

To not participate.

Orlando sat out the discussion portion of the Alcoholics Anonymous meeting because he wasn't comfortable sharing his feelings with the other attendees.

Sit tight

To wait.

The doctor told the patient he would just have to sit tight and see if the medication worked.

Sit up and take notice

To show interest.

The patient didn't sit up and take notice of the doctor's orders until she told him that he would die if he didn't quit smoking.

Sitting on a powder keg

To be in a very risky or potentially volatile situation.

When the nurses threatened to go on strike, the hospital administrators knew that they were sitting on a powder keg.

Sitting pretty

To be well situated.

If the patient's cancer stays in remission for five

years, she will be sitting pretty in terms of making a full recovery.

Six of one, half a dozen of the other

About the same.

Generic and brand name drugs are virtually identical, so when choosing between them, it is six of one, half a dozen of the other.

Skate on thin ice

To be in a precarious situation.

If the patient does not comply with his treatment he will be skating on thin ice.

Skeleton in (one's) closet

A hidden secret.

The patient found it difficult to reveal the skeletons in his closet to his therapist.

Skin and bones

Very thin.

The anorexic woman was nothing but skin and bones.

Skin (someone) alive

To punish someone severely.

The nurse threatened to skin the intern alive if he disturbed the ICU patient.

Sky rocket

To take off quickly.

The idea for the new physical therapy rehab clinic really sky rocketed with the orthopedic department's total support.

Slack off

To diminish or taper off; *also*, to be lazy.

At first, Jean experienced some unpleasant side effects to the new medication, but they slacked off in just a few days.

Slap in the face

An insult.

When the hospital administrators denied their request for a departmental salary increase, the nursing staff considered it a slap in the face.

Slated for (something)

Scheduled for something.

The patient is slated for surgery tomorrow.

Sleep in

To sleep past one's normal wake-up time.

Mario needed lots of rest in order to recover from the flu, so Dr. Sams encouraged him to take a few days off work and sleep in.

Sleep like a log *or* Sleep like a baby

To sleep very deeply.

The naturopathic doctor told Doreen that taking melatonin supplements would help her sleep like a baby.

Sleep on it

To think something over before making a decision.

The patient did not know what course of action to take, so he told Dr. Vasser he would sleep on it.

Slip of the tongue

To speak inappropriately.

The nurse didn't mean to criticize the doctor's decision; it was a slip of the tongue.

Slow on the uptake

Not able to process ideas quickly.

The head nurse recommended that Layla be transferred out of the emergency department, because she tended to be slow on the uptake.

Slowly but surely

To succeed gradually.

Slowly but surely, the physical therapy sessions helped Terrence regain the use of his arm.

Smack-dab in the middle

Right in the center.

The boy needed stitches smack-dab in the middle of his forehead.

Small hours of the night

Hours immediately after midnight.

It seems most babies are born in the small hours of the night.

Small-time

Modest.

Before taking the chief of staff position at the hospital, Dr. Stahl had a small-time clinic in the suburbs.

Smoke and mirrors

Deceptive and confusing.

Georgia worried that her insurance company's explanation of benefits forms was nothing but smoke and mirrors.

Smooth sailing

Progress made without any difficulty.

After the initial crisis passed, it was smooth sailing, and the patient made steady improvement.

Snake in the grass

A deceitful person.

Paul switched primary care physicians, saying that his former doctor was a snake in the grass.

Snap out of (something)

To become suddenly freed from a state or condition.

My colds usually last for a week or two, but this time I snapped out of it in just a few days.

Snug as a bug in a rug

Cozy.

The pediatric nurses always tuck the small patients in at night, making sure each one is snug as a bug in a rug.

So be it

Then that is the way it will be.

If the patient refuses chemotherapy, so be it.

So far, so good

Things are proceeding without difficulty.

Caden asked how his treatment course was going, and the doctor told him so far, so good.

So much the better

Even better.

If the patient can add an additional 10 minutes to his therapy session, so much the better.

So quiet you can hear a pin drop

A state of complete silence.

When the doctor gave Earl his prognosis, the room was so quiet you could hear a pin drop.

So to speak

As one might say.

Polly is so enthusiastic and supportive at the hospital's intramural softball games, she's become the head cheerleader, so to speak.

Solid as a rock

Very dependable.

The expansion plan submitted to the Board of Directors is solid as a rock, and there should be no trouble getting it approved.

(Someone) just doesn't get it

An inability to relate to or understand someone or something.

I tried to explain the HIPAA regulations to Mary Beth several times, but she just doesn't get it.

Something to that effect

Something similar to that.

Dr. Souders told Clarissa to exercise by walking, swimming, or something to that effect.

Something's up

Acknowledging that things are out of the ordinary and that something unusual is happening or going to happen.

Something's up: Dr. Dean is in a hurry to get Mr. Harold's test results.

Sound like a broken record

To repeat the same thing over and over.

Perry is starting to sound like a broken record with all his complaints about the workload in the emergency department.

Space out

To become incoherent or unfocused.

The patient was completely spaced out when he came into the hospital and was immediately admitted for a drug overdose.

Spaz out

To become extremely agitated; spastic.

Beverly will spaz out if the nurse doesn't bring her medications on time.

Speak of the devil

To refer to someone who has just arrived.

Speak of the devil, here comes Robbie now.

Speak out

To make one's opinion known.

At the board meeting, Yolanda decided to speak out against the patient privacy violations occurring at the hospital.

Speak out of turn

To say something inappropriate.

Even if she did speak out of turn, Jada felt it was right to let the patient know his prognosis.

Speak up

To come forward and state one's opinion.

If you feel the therapist's comments are not appropriate, you must speak up.

Spell (something) out

To be very explicit.

The doctor carefully spelled all the instructions out for the patient.

Spic and span

Exceptionally clean.

The hospital has to ensure that each patient's room is spic and span.

Split hairs

To argue over something insignificant or petty.

Even though she preferred the brand name drug, Adelle didn't want to split hairs with the pharmacist, so she took the generic.

Spoon-feed (someone)

To give someone too much assistance.

The new residents quickly learned that the doctors did not have time to spoon-feed them.

Spread like wildfire

To expand rapidly.

The patient stated that the rash spread like wildfire.

Square peg in a round hole

Ill-fitting.

Edith is so active that putting her in a nursing home would be like trying to fit a square peg in a round hole.

Stack the cards *or* Stack the deck

To arrange circumstances in a way that will produce a particular end result.

When Marsha heard that there was an opportunity for one of the night-shift attendants to move to the day shift, she tried to stack the cards in her favor by flattering her superiors and bringing them home-baked goodies.

Stand corrected

To admit one is wrong.

Although I told you the test results would be in today, I stand corrected: They won't be ready until tomorrow.

Stand for (something)

To allow something to occur; *also*, to represent a particular cause.

The ICU nurse is very strict and will not stand for noise or commotion in the hallways.

Stand in awe

To be overwhelmed with respect for someone or something.

I couldn't help but stand in awe of the president of AAMT when I met her.

Stand in for (something or someone)

To act as a substitute.

Dr. Rudolph stood in for Dr. Weston and did his rounds for him while he was on vacation.

Stand to reason

To seem reasonable.

It stands to reason that if you ignore the doctor's orders, your condition won't improve.

Stark raving mad

Insane.

When she stopped taking her antipsychotic medication, the patient went stark raving mad.

Start from scratch

To begin with nothing.

After a three-month lapse, the patient had to start from scratch on his rehab.

Start off on the wrong foot

To get off to a bad beginning.

Mr. Huot arrived half an hour early for his new job at the clinic, as he didn't want to start off on the wrong foot.

Start the ball rolling

To initiate something.

Dr. Ling wanted to start the ball rolling by setting specific goals for the patient so they could best determine the course of action.

Start with a clean slate

To have a fresh beginning.

Jermaine was eager to start with a clean slate after completing his drug rehab program.

Steer clear

To avoid something or someone.

The doctor was careful with his dosage recommendations of the medication because he wanted to steer clear of any complications.

Step-by-step

Detailed.

Elena needed step-by-step instructions on how to use the Thera-Band.

Step down

To resign.

The doctor stepped down to allow the consultant to take over the patient's care.

Step on the gas

To hurry.

The frantic accident victim told the 911 operator to have the paramedics step on the gas.

Stick in the mud

A boring person.

When he advised her to stop drinking and smoking, Anna called Dr. Franklin a stick in the mud.

Stick out like a sore thumb

To be obviously out of place.

As the only male on the nursing staff, Ned sticks out like a sore thumb.

Stir up a hornet's nest

To provoke an attack; to create a problem.

The radical Patients' Rights group was just trying to stir up a hornet's nest by reporting grossly inflated numbers of accidental hospital deaths.

Stop at nothing

To do everything possible to accomplish a goal.

Marsha would stop at nothing to get her son the best possible treatment for his leukemia.

Stop, look, and listen

To exercise caution.

When crossing the street, be sure you stop, look, and listen.

Straight and narrow

A responsible course of action.

When he suffered a setback due to his own actions, Ollie vowed to go on the straight and narrow, following his doctor's orders precisely.

Straight from the horse's mouth

To receive information from the original source.

It is true that Mindy is pregnant: I heard it straight from the horse's mouth.

Strictly on the up-and-up

Ethical, legal, and honest.

Nathan wasn't sure that the HMO's billing procedures were strictly on the up-and-up.

Strike a balance

To find a satisfactory compromise between two extremes.

Striking a balance between overdosing and underdosing the new medication has been a challenge for researchers.

Strike a happy medium

To compromise.

The committee was able to strike a happy medium on the issue of the new quality standards.

Strike up a conversation

To begin talking to someone.

The two women struck up a conversation in the clinic waiting room.

Strung out

Extended over a period of time or large space; *also,* altered behavior brought on by a chemical substance.

The patient was brought into the emergency department in labor and strung out on heroin.

Stubborn as a mule

Obstinate.

Sometimes Lorna is as stubborn as a mule and refuses to do the exercises her physical therapist recommends.

Subject (someone) to (something)

To inflict something on someone.

When she volunteered for the study, Nessa knew she would be subjected to numerous questions regarding her experiences and reactions to the medication the researchers were investigating.

Such as

To resemble or exemplify.

The doctor wanted the patient to adopt an exercise program, such as walking three times a week and swimming two days a week.

Supply and demand

The availability of services or merchandise in contrast to the number of customers who desire it.

Whether or not the rehab clinic will remain in operation will depend on supply and demand, so the more referrals they get, the more likely they are to stay open.

Survival of the fittest

The idea that the strongest members of a group will succeed while the weakest will fail.

Medical residency is so demanding that it comes

down to survival of the fittest in order to determine who makes it and who doesn't.

Swallow (something) hook, line, and sinker

To believe something that is untrue.

Vivian is so gullible: She swallowed the patient's story hook, line, and sinker.

Sweep (something) under the rug

To hide something unpleasant.

Mel had a tendency to sweep his problems under the rug rather than openly discussing them with the doctor.

Swift and sure

Quickly and with certainty.

The surgeon opened the patient's chest with one incision, made swift and sure.

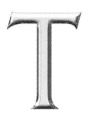

T

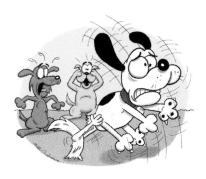

Tail wagging the dog

24-7

All the time; 24 hours a day, 7 days a week.

Working as the chief radiologist for Memorial Hospital's emergency department, Dr. Gulding needs to be available 24-7.

Tail wagging the dog

A small part of something controlling the overall entity.

Pharmaceutical companies would like more control in the FDA's drug approval process, but that would be like the tail wagging the dog.

Take a backseat to (someone or something)

To become inferior to someone or something else.

When the patient went into cardiac arrest, setting his broken leg took a backseat to resuscitating him.

Take a crack at (something)

To try something.

Even after discussing it with the surgeon, Mitch was still reticent to have surgery, so the resident decided to take a crack at convincing him it was the right thing to do.

Take a dim view of (something)

To regard something with reservation, skepticism, or disapproval.

Geo knew that if he couldn't quit smoking, his doctor would take a dim view of his commitment to become healthier.

Take a gander

To examine someone or something.

The doctor will take a gander at the x-rays to see if there are any abnormalities.

Take a hard line

To be very firm with someone.

Dr. Rodgers took a hard line with Tom because he hadn't been taking the full dose of Coumadin she prescribed to him.

Take a hike

Go away.

After two weeks under constant surveillance by the nursing staff, Preston wished they would take a hike and give him some privacy.

Take a load off

To sit down and rest.

Before they began the second half of their session, the physical therapist invited Carly to take a load off for a few minutes.

Take a long walk off a short pier

Go away.

Barbara lost her patience with Dr. Zelman and told him to take a long walk off a short pier.

Take a rain check

To decline a scheduled event but request that it take place in the future.

Ned was invited to stay for dinner, but said he had to take a rain check because he had made other plans for the evening.

Take a spill

To fall.

The paramedics rushed Mr. Hathaway to the ED after he took a spill down the stairs of his home.

Take a stab at (something)

To make an attempt to do something.

Marcia wasn't sure if she had regained full use of her hand after her reconstructive surgery, but she decided to take a stab at playing the piano anyway.

Take a turn for the better

To improve.

The patient took a turn for the better after he began taking the antibiotic his doctor prescribed.

Take a turn for the worse

To deteriorate.

Despite all efforts, the patient took a turn for the worse.

Take advantage of (someone or something)

To use something or someone for one's own benefit.

Mary took advantage of the insurance company's mail-order prescription drug program.

Take effect

To become effective.

The law will take effect at noon tomorrow.

Take exception to (something)

To take offense to or disagree with something.

Enzo believes that the health benefits of red wine outweigh any potential risks, so he took exception to his doctor's advice that he give up alcohol altogether.

Take five

To take a short break.

After running on the treadmill for 20 minutes, Lance asked his doctor if he could take five before he continued with his stress test.

Take great pains to (do something)

To put forth substantial effort to accomplish something.

Laurel took great pains to make sure she completed the project on time.

Take heart

To have courage or confidence.

When Millie got discouraged with her slow recovery process, Dr. Chan told her to take heart because her overall prognosis was good.

Take it easy

To relax and enjoy oneself; *also*, to be gentle.

Dr. Eisenberg told the resident to take it easy when helping elderly patients into wheelchairs, since their bones can be very brittle.

Take it or leave it

To be given the choice to either accept an offer or reject it.

Julie told the patient she could give him extra thera-

py after 6 p.m. He wasn't sure he wanted to do that, but she told him to take it or leave it.

Take leave of (one's) senses

To act, speak, or think irrationally.

Sandra must have taken leave of her senses when she walked through the city barefoot: Now she has a serious fungal infection.

Take note of (something)

To notice something.

The psychiatrist took note of the patient's physical tics in addition to his emotional problems.

Take off

To leave.

The geriatric ward staff has to keep an eye on Mr. Pena, because he tends to take off and wander the halls.

Take (one) at (one's) word

To believe what someone says.

I will take you at your word that you took all the medication prescribed.

Take (one's) cue from (something)

To proceed based on the results of something else.

We will take our cue from the patient's reaction to the new drug regimen, and then determine whether or not additional measures are necessary.

Take part in (something)

To participate.

Dr. Moore asked one of the interns to take part in Kaleb's physical exam.

Take sick

To become ill.

Maggie told the doctor she took sick two days ago.

Take some getting used to

A significant change that requires a period of adjustment.

Being on a new medication regimen may take some getting used to.

Take (someone) down a notch or two

To humble someone who is overly confident.

Doug thought he could handle his alcohol addiction on his own, but when he suffered a relapse it took him down a notch or two and he finally sought help.

Take (someone) for a ride

To trick or deceive someone.

The addict tried to take his counselor for a ride, denying that he'd used drugs the previous day.

Take (someone's) breath away

To shock someone.

Casey told the doctor that the pain in her side was enough to take her breath away.

Take (someone's) pulse

To measure someone's heart rate.

When the patient arrived at the hospital, the nurse took her pulse before checking her other vital signs.

Take (something) at face value

To accept something as it is.

The doctor took Gloria's complaints at face value and prescribed her a pain reliever without giving her a full exam.

Take (something) in stride

To accept an unpleasant or inconvenient occurrence without concern.

The young boy seemed to take his broken arm in stride and even enjoyed having his friends sign his cast.

Take (something) with a grain of salt

To regard something with skepticism.

Renee took her fatigue with a grain of salt, but Dr. Abrams thought it might be a symptom of hypothyroidism.

Take the bull by the horns

To face a challenge without fear.

Paul knew that in order to regain full use of his legs, he would have to take the bull by the horns and begin daily physical therapy sessions.

Take the liberty of (doing something)

To make a decision or take an action that requires someone else's permission or approval without consulting them about it.

Shawn took the liberty of increasing his dose of Paxil without his psychiatrist's approval.

Take the trouble

To perform a tedious or bothersome task.

The nurses always take the trouble to bring patients pitchers of water or extra pillows.

Take the wind out of (someone's) sails

To ruin someone's good mood.

When Dr. LeBroc told Jerry that he hadn't made adequate progress after three months on the new drug regimen, it definitely took the wind out of his sails.

Talk a blue streak

To talk a lot.

The activities director quickly discovered that many of the elderly patients can talk a blue streak.

Talk in circles

To discuss something without ever arriving at the main point.

The drug counselor found that many rehab patients talk in circles to avoid accepting responsibility for their actions.

Tamper with (something)

To alter something.

The lab technician feared that someone had tampered with the urine sample, causing the test results to be unreliable.

Tar and feather

To punish someone severely.

Dr. Lester threatened to tar and feather Olive if she continued to eat fried foods.

Team up

To collaborate.

The speech therapist will team up with the rehab therapist to assist the patient's recovery.

Tee (someone) off

To make someone angry or upset.

Gretchen got teed off when the doctor cancelled her appointment at the last minute.

Tell tales out of school

To spread rumors.

When the hospital chief-of-staff found out that one of the nurses had been gossiping with patients about the doctors' private lives, he warned her not to tell tales out of school.

Tell which is which

To distinguish a difference between two things.

The patient complained of blurred vision, but when asked which eye was worse, he could not tell which was which.

Tempest in a teapot

Someone who makes a fuss over something unimportant.

Janet reacted like a tempest in a teapot over Mike's sprained ankle when his real problem was a serious concussion.

That does it!

An exclamation in reference to a catalyst that brings someone to action.

That does it! If the insurance company denies one more of my claims, I am going to cancel my coverage.

That takes care of that

That settles the matter.

The doctor told JoAnn than she had no choice but to undergo bypass surgery, so that takes care of that.

That's all she wrote

There is nothing more to do or say; we're done.

When Elaine finished her x-rays, the radiologist said, "That's all she wrote," and told her she could go home.

That's the way the ball bounces

A statement acknowledging that an occurrence has happened for a reason.

When Adam suffered a relapse because he didn't take his medication, the doctor told him that that's the way the ball bounces.

That's the way the cookie crumbles

A statement acknowledging that an occurrence has happened for a reason.

Mack didn't think that forgetting to take his medication for one day would affect him, but he had a serious reaction, and his doctor told him that that's the way the cookie crumbles.

The bottom line

The final outcome.

The patient has not responded to treatment, so the bottom line is that he will need surgery.

The coast is clear

No trouble is in sight.

After a few minor side effects, the patient had no further complications to the treatment protocol, so the doctor said it looked like the coast was clear.

The daily grind

The regular routine.

After a lengthy stay in rehab, many drug addicts find it difficult to readjust to the daily grind without resorting back to substance abuse.

The here and now

The present.

Although her case of pancreatic cancer has been diagnosed as terminal, Lenora continues to live for the here and now, enjoying as many of her usual activities as she can.

The inside track

An advantageous position due to special connections.

The other insurance carrier had the inside track with the company's CEO, so they received the contract.

The jig is up

The deception is over.

When her doctor noticed that she hadn't lost any weight since her last visit, Marcy knew that the jig was up and she'd have to start following his diet recommendations.

The jury is still out

A final decision has not yet been made.

The doctors can't decide whether or not the patient will need surgery; the jury is still out on that one.

The last straw

A final negative incident that prompts corrective action.

When Baltimore Oriole's pitcher Steve Bechler died after taking ephedra, it was the last straw in prompting the FDA to ban the product from the market.

The more the merrier

The greater the number of people involved in an activity, the more enjoyable it will be.

The young couple wanted as many friends and family members as possible to attend the birth of their first baby, telling them the more the merrier.

The other way around

The opposite.

Terri thought the new drug would cure her arthritis symptoms, but it ended up being the other way around: It only increased her pain and inflammation.

The pits

The worst possible situation.

Most children think that taking medicine is the pits.

The pot calling the kettle black

To accuse someone of something that the accuser himself does.

Dr. Frost admonished Lucy for not getting enough sleep, but that was the pot calling the kettle black.

The shoe is on the other foot

To experience the same thing that one had caused others to experience.

Dr. Palmer has advised hundreds of patients to take statin drugs to lower their cholesterol, but now that his own doctor has prescribed them to him, the shoe is on the other foot.

The sky is the limit

The possibilities are endless.

Jorg's physician told him that the sky is the limit as to how much improvement he could expect from the new treatment protocol.

The straw that broke the camel's back

A final negative incident that prompts corrective action.

George's continued noncompliance was the straw that broke the camel's back and his mom enrolled him in a group therapy class.

The works

To receive everything available.

When you get a full body massage, you get the works.

There aren't enough hours in the day

There is too little time.

The residents were overworked and told their supervisor that there simply weren't enough hours in the day to complete all of their assigned tasks.

There's more than one way to skin a cat

There are numerous ways to accomplish something.

Ethel's doctor told her that there's more than one way to skin a cat and gave her several options for alleviating her sciatica pain.

Thick-skinned

Not easily offended.

Serving on the board of directors makes you thick-skinned: You learn not to take criticism personally.

Thin-skinned

Easily offended.

Zena tends to be thin-skinned, so her counselor tried to phrase his recommendations as delicately as possible.

Think back

To remember.

The doctor asked the patient to think back to when her symptoms actually started.

Think highly of (someone or something)

Regard something with much favor.

The hospital board thinks very highly of Dr. Scott because he attends to each of his patients with the utmost care and professionalism.

Think on (one's) feet

To act quickly and decisively.

Working in the emergency department forces doctors and nurses to think on their feet.

Think outside the box

To consider untraditional ideas or approaches.

Sometimes therapists must think outside the box to find new, creative ways to rehabilitate patients.

Think (something) out

To consider all aspects of an issue thoroughly.

Josephine repeatedly asked the doctor to think out her various treatment options before she resigned herself to surgery.

Think twice

To reconsider something.

Dr. Wesley warned Sophie to think twice before quitting her medication because she could suffer serious withdrawal symptoms.

Three sheets to the wind

Intoxicated.

The patient was three sheets to the wind when the EMTs arrived at the scene.

Through thick and thin

During good times and bad.

Darlene's husband was by her side during the whole course of her cancer, through thick and thin.

Throw caution to the wind

To act carelessly or recklessly.

After many months of intense physical therapy, Betty was ready to throw caution to the wind and get rid of her walker.

Throw in the towel

To give up.

After multiple failed attempts at in vitro fertiliza-tion, the couple decided to throw in the towel and look into adopting a child instead.

Throw (someone) a curve *or* Throw (someone) a curve ball

To surprise someone by doing something that is unex-pected.

The unexpected effects of the drug threw the re-searchers a curve.

Tied up

Busy.

Dr. Otis has been tied up with patient emergencies all morning and hasn't been able to check his messages.

Time after time

Repeatedly.

I have told you time after time, if you don't know how to take a medication, call the doctor or phar-macist for help.

Time will tell

The answer will become apparent in time.

So far, studies have only been done on rats: Only time will tell if the new drug's effects can be dupli-cated in humans.

To a great extent

Primarily.

To a great extent, doctors rely on pharmaceutical drugs to treat their patients.

To put it mildly

To understate something.

The state of healthcare in the United States frustrates many people, to put it mildly.

Tongue-in-cheek

In jest; teasing.

Mark made a tongue-in-cheek comment to Dr. Lang about his bedside manner.

Too good to be true

Something so positive it is almost unbelievable.

When Julie's doctor told her about an experimental drug that might cure her psoriasis, she thought it sounded too good to be true.

Too much of a good thing

More of something than is appropriate.

Beth's nutritionist told her that, in moderation, red wine has valuable health benefits, but warned her not to drink it in excess, since too much of a good thing can have negative consequences.

Touch and go

Uncertain; precarious.

The patient's condition was touch and go for a while.

Touch base

To get in contact with someone.

The patient's doctor encouraged her to touch base with him on a regular basis to update him on her status.

Tough nut to crack

A difficult person or thing to figure out.

Though we've run just about every available test, this is really a tough nut to crack. We're still unable to determine what is causing the patient's symptoms.

Tough row to hoe

Something difficult to undertake.

Learning medical transcription is a tough row to hoe.

Tower of strength

An extremely dependable person.

Raul was a tower of strength to Zach's family during Zach's illness.

Train of thought

Pattern of thinking.

Dr. Manning lost his train of thought when the nurse knocked on the exam room door.

Trial and error

A process of discovering something that involves many failed attempts before arriving at the final outcome.

The pharmaceutical research and development team created the new formula for the drug through trial and error.

Trick or treat!

A saying used on Halloween, an American holiday on which children go from house to house collecting candy.

When I opened the door, the children cried, "Trick or treat!"

Tricks of the trade

The knowledge that is necessary to be an expert in one's field.

After 10 years as a pharmaceutical representative, Josie has learned all the tricks of the trade and can sell a new drug to just about anyone.

Tried and true

Reliable.

Although there are many new drugs available to treat arthritis, a lot of doctors still recommend acetaminophen because it is tried and true.

Turn in

Go to bed.

Dr. Appleton decided to turn in early since he had to report back to the hospital by 5:00 the next morning.

Turn the tide

To change the course of something.

Increasing the patient's dose of antibiotics turned the tide in his condition and he made a full recovery within a week.

Turn up the heat

To put pressure on someone or something.

The hospital had to turn up the heat on the insurance company to get it to cover the patient's surgical procedure.

Two's company but three's a crowd

Sometimes it is better to have less people involved in something; often shortened to "three's a crowd."

The obstetrician told the couple to think carefully before inviting a lot of people into the delivery room to witness their baby's birth, saying that two's company but three's a crowd.

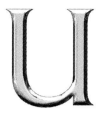

U

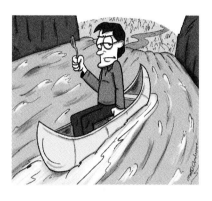

*Up the creek
without a paddle*

Under a cloud of suspicion

To be suspected of doing something.

When Dr. Richards determined that the patient's complications resulted from him receiving the wrong medication, everyone on the previous shift was under a cloud of suspicion.

Under fire

To be scrutinized or attacked.

The hospital administrator came under fire from the insurance companies for allowing the patient to stay longer than the diagnosis dictated.

Under scrutiny

To be examined or watched closely.

The methodology of the exam came under scrutiny after several patients sustained injury.

Under the auspices of (someone or something)

Subject to the control, monitoring, supervision, or sponsorship of someone or something.

The new CT scanner is under the auspices of the Radiology Department.

Under the circumstances

Based on a specific situation or occurrence.

The patient's condition weakened considerably, so, under the circumstances, the doctor gave strict orders that she was not to be moved.

Under the counter *or* Under the table

Obtained from an illegal source or in an illegal manner.

Steve's overdose occurred after he took some drugs he got under the counter.

Under the influence

To have one's normal functioning be impaired by alcohol, chemicals, or a controlling individual.

The EMTs reported that the patient's motor vehicle accident occurred while she was under the influence of alcohol.

Under the sun

Anywhere on Earth.

All of the failed treatment attempts Brandon endured convinced him that nothing under the sun could help him.

Under the weather

Not healthy.

The patient complained of feeling a little under the weather.

Until all hours of the night

Very late.

The young mother looked exhausted and admitted to the pediatrician that the baby had kept her up until all hours of the night.

Until hell freezes over

Forever.

Milo vowed not to give up fighting his cancer until hell freezes over.

Until the cows come home

For a very long time.

Bev is convinced that she can diet and exercise until the cows come home and still not lose any weight.

Up a tree

In a difficult situation without any way out.

Damian was up a tree when he had an asthma attack and realized that he didn't have his inhaler.

Up against (something)

To be faced with a problem or threat.

The patient is up against a serious staph infection and will have a very hard time fighting it without the proper medication.

Up and about *or* Up and around

Out of bed and moving around.

The doctor told Fran that she could be up and about as much as she could tolerate.

Up and at 'em

Awake and busy.

Residents are used to being up and at 'em very early in the morning.

Up-and-coming

New and innovative.

The up-and-coming pharmaceutical company just released two brand new drugs.

Up for grabs

Available to anyone.

When Luther was discharged from the hospital, the private room he'd been in went up for grabs.

Up in years

Elderly.

The patient was getting up in years and couldn't perform her daily activities as well as she used to.

Up the creek without a paddle

In a hopeless situation.

Because of his serious allergy, Jesse must take every precaution to avoid eating peanuts; otherwise he will be up the creek without a paddle.

Up to date

Current or modern.

Dr. Moore wanted to wait for more up-to-date research on the drug before prescribing it to his patients.

Up to no good

Behaving badly.

The rehab counselor could tell that several of the inpatients were up to no good just by the looks on their faces.

Up to (one's) neck *or* Up to (one's) eyeballs *or* Up to (one's) ears

To have an excess of something.

Jamie has so many prescriptions she feels like she's up to her neck in pills every day.

Up to par

Meeting the established standards.

The new drug is up to par with the others in its category.

Up to snuff

To meet the expected standard.

Even though the patient was trying to add additional repetitions to his program, he was just not up to snuff today.

Up-to-the-minute

The latest or most recent.

The doctor wanted up-to-the-minute reports on the patient's condition.

Ups and downs

Good and bad aspects.

Chemotherapy has its ups and downs, but with so few other treatment options for cancer, it is usually worth trying.

Upset the apple cart

To cause a disturbance.

Suzanne Somers upset the apple cart when she chose to forgo mainstream treatment options and adopt a complimentary medicine approach to treating her breast cancer instead.

Use every trick in the book

To employ every possible technique to do something.

The patient used every trick in the book to get more Prozac.

Use some elbow grease

To put physical effort into something.

The EMTs had to use some elbow grease to lift the 400-pound man into the ambulance.

Use (someone or something) as an excuse

To blame someone or something as a reason for doing something inappropriate.

Nora used her hypoglycemia as an excuse to eat several candy bars a day.

Use strong language

To swear or verbally threaten.

Without her medication, the patient became agitated and began using strong language.

Use your noggin *or* Use your noodle *or* Use your head

Think.

The doctor told Patty to use her noggin and base her diet on common sense instead of fads.

Used to (something or someone)

To be familiar with or accustomed to something or someone.

The patient had a hard time getting used to the new protocol.

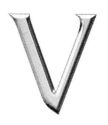

V

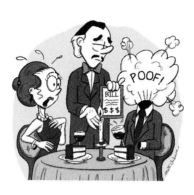

Vanish into thin air

Vanish into thin air

To disappear.

James said that after just three days on the new antiinflammatory drug, his arthritis pain vanished into thin air.

Variety is the spice of life

Life is made interesting by trying and doing different things.

Kevin's physical therapist told him that variety is the spice of life and recommended that he alternate his exercise regimen between jogging, swimming, and cycling.

Verge of (something)

To be very close to doing something.

Scientists are on the verge of discovering a cure for the common cold.

Very thing

Exactly what is needed at the moment.

Rest is the very thing I need right now.

Vim and vigor

Energy and enthusiasm.

Now that he has fully recovered from the injuries he sustained in the car accident, Reese is full of vim and vigor.

Vote a split ticket

To cast a ballot in which votes are divided between two parties.

Terri could not decide which party to vote for, so she voted a split ticket.

Vote a straight ticket

To cast a ballot with all votes for members of the same political party.

I always vote a straight ticket because I believe in the principles of the party.

Vote of confidence

To support someone or something.

Rachel felt better about taking the drug when her doctor told her it had his vote of confidence.

Vote of thanks

Recognition from a group for a job well done.

Kim was given a vote of thanks for her extraordinary dedication to the new Women's Care wing.

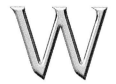

W

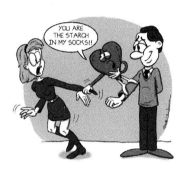

*Wear your heart
on your sleeve*

Wait-and-see attitude

To approach a problem without urgency.

The doctor had a wait-and-see attitude about the patient's progress.

Wait in the wings

To be ready or willing to do something.

Dr. West was the primary care physician for the patient, but Dr. Olson was waiting in the wings to assist.

Wait on (someone) hand and foot

To attend to someone's every need.

Mason expected the nurse to wait on him hand and foot.

Wait up

To delay going to bed in anticipation of something else.

Bill's wife waited up until she got a call from Bill's surgeon saying that the procedure had gone well.

Walk a tightrope

To be in a very tense situation.

ICU and ED physicians walk a tightrope every day, trying to save the lives of patients in critical condition.

Walk off with (something)

To take or steal something.

May's doctor gave her so many free samples that she walked off with a six-month supply of her prescription blood pressure medication.

Walk on eggshells

To act or speak very cautiously.

The new head resident had such a bad temper that all of the other residents felt they had to walk on eggshells when they were around him.

Walk the floor

To pace around a room.

Most fathers-to-be spend a lot of time walking the floor in the maternity ward waiting room while their wives are in labor.

Walls have ears

To be overheard by someone whom you cannot see.

The pharmaceutical company representative told Dr. King that the walls have ears, so he couldn't reveal any of the details about the new drug until the formula received a patent.

Want for nothing

To possess everything one needs.

The Ramos family does not have a lot of money, but they seem to want for nothing.

Wash (one's) hands of (something or someone)

To end a relationship with someone or to distance one-self from a situation.

Dr. Gladstone warned Veronica that if she didn't comply with the prescribed treatment and chose to put herself at risk instead, he would wash his hands of her.

Watch (someone) like a hawk

To pay close attention to someone.

The maternity ward nurse watched the fetal heart monitor like a hawk, looking for any signs of trouble.

Wax and wane

To increase and decrease.

The patient said that his pain waxed and waned.

Way of life

Lifestyle.

Emergency department physicians work so many late-night and early-morning shifts that lack of sleep usually becomes a way of life.

Ways and means

Funds and procedures used to attain something.

The advisory panel discussed the ways and means by which the hospital could attain the equipment necessary to provide its patients with optimal care.

Weak as a kitten

Sickly and fatigued.

Helena complained that she felt weak as a kitten and could barely climb the stairs in her house.

Wear and tear

The natural process of breaking down or deteriorating that occurs when something is used regularly.

Wear and tear on the joints can result in osteoarthritis.

Wear more than one hat

To have more than one job, or to have many different responsibilities.

Steve wears more than one hat at the hospital: He is an administrator and a HIPAA privacy officer.

Wear (one's) heart on (one's) sleeve

To openly display one's feelings.

Everyone knows how much Dr. Soo cares for her patients because she wears her heart on her sleeve.

Wear out (one's) welcome

To stay too long.

Hospital visiting hour regulations are intended to keep patients' friends and relatives from wearing out their welcome.

Wear (someone) down

To overcome someone by persistent verbal persuasion.

Carl resisted cutting back on salt, but his cardiologist finally wore him down, and he finally agreed to use a salt substitute instead.

Weather permitting

Assuming the weather is nice.

Weather permitting, we will have the hospital staff picnic tomorrow.

Wee hours of the morning

Very early.

Kristy's sister called today to announce that her niece had been born in the wee hours of the morning.

Wee hours of the night

Hours immediately after midnight.

Andraya was up until the wee hours of the night trying to comfort the newborn.

Week in and week out

Continually.

Paulette became bored with her physical therapy regimen after just two months because she felt as if she was doing the same exercises week in and week out.

Weigh on (one's) mind

To be burdened or preoccupied with something.

Dr. Alderman lets his patients' problems weigh on his mind so much that he cannot relax when he gets home.

Well off

Wealthy.

Most people think that all doctors are rich, but many are not as well off as you might think.

Well to do

Wealthy.

Josh did not have to worry about paying for medical school because his family is well to do.

Wet behind the ears

Inexperienced.

Mildred was nervous about letting the young resi-dent treat her, since he was still wet behind the ears.

Wet blanket

A dull or negative person.

When her usual primary care doctor couldn't see her, Dora hoped she wouldn't have to see Dr. Dalton instead: She thinks he is a wet blanket.

What are you driving at?

To ask someone about the point of their questions or statements.

The doctor questioned Nicolas at length about his social habits, so Nicolas finally asked her what she was driving at.

What goes around comes around

One's good or bad behaviors and actions will be repaid eventually.

Rebeka has always been supportive and giving, and when she was in a crisis, her friends and family were there for her. It just goes to show that what goes around comes around.

What has (one) been up to?

To question someone about their recent activities.

Dr. Jamison asked Stella what she'd been up to since her last appointment.

What if

To wonder about the possible outcome that might result from a particular incident or decision.

What if you had not gotten to the hospital in time?

What is keeping (someone)

A reason for someone's tardiness.

When he was 45 minutes late for their appointment, Evelyn wondered what was keeping Dr. Wendel.

When all is said and done

To reach a point of completion.

When all is said and done, the patient really has made every effort to control her blood sugar.

When hell freezes over

Never.

Antoni vowed that he would stop fighting his cancer when hell freezes over.

When in Rome, do as the Romans

Conduct oneself in the same manner as those around you.

All of the clinic's inpatients meditated before bed each night, so Muriel thought, "When in Rome, do as the Romans," and tried meditation herself.

When it comes right down to it

When you consider the very core of the issue.

When it comes right down to it, if you do not exercise, you will not stay in shape.

When it rains, it pours

Said when several bad things occur at the same time.

In a single week, Sydney's husband fell, her daughter broke her arm, and her son needed stitches. When it rains, it pours.

When least expected

To be unprepared for an occurrence.

Many people report that their GERD and heartburn flare-ups seem to occur when least expected.

When push comes to shove

When a situation becomes critical.

When push comes to shove, all the departments work together to get the job done.

When the chips are down

A bad or desperate situation.

Valerie took a job in the free clinic so that she could help people when the chips are down.

When the going gets tough, the tough get going

Acts of perseverance and strength displayed during a very difficult situation.

EMTs that responded to the 9/11 disaster in New York encountered an overwhelming number of peo-

ple with severe injuries, but when the going gets tough, the tough get going.

Where there's a will, there's a way

Determination that drives someone to accomplish a goal.

After his accident, Christopher was convinced that he would walk again someday. He believes that where there's a will, there's a way.

Whip (something) up

To create or prepare something in a short period of time.

The pharmaceutical company's research and development team whipped up six new drug formulations.

White as a sheet

Extremely pale.

When the patient went into shock, her face turned white as a sheet.

Who do you think you are kidding?

To question someone regarding their attempt to deceive or hide something from someone.

Even though Jan insisted that she had followed his recommendations perfectly, Dr. Remus could tell from her test results that she hadn't, so he asked, "Who do you think you are kidding?"

Who would have thought?

To comment on an unexpected outcome of a situation.

Who would have thought that the patient's heart would start beating again 20 minutes after he'd flatlined.

Whole ball of wax

Something in its entirety.

Brian listed his symptoms for Dr. Xavier and told him that was the whole ball of wax.

Whole kit and caboodle

The whole thing.

The visiting nurse arrived with the whole kit and caboodle of everything she needed to take care of the patient.

Whole new ball game *or* Whole different ball game

An entirely different set of circumstances.

With Dr. Kenney in charge, doing rounds became a whole new ball game.

Whys and wherefores

The reasons for something.

Dr. Fawcett told Zoe not to worry about the whys and wherefores of her condition, but to focus instead on her recovery.

Wild goose chase

A complicated or futile course of action.

Trying to track down the origin of the SARS outbreak led researchers on a wild goose chase.

Wild horses couldn't drag (someone) (somewhere)

To refuse to do something regardless of external influence or pressure.

Sharon does not like hospitals, and she says wild horses couldn't drag her there.

Wind down

To decrease or diminish.

The ER was very busy tonight, but things are beginning to wind down.

Window shopping

To look at something but not buy it.

Susan doesn't have much money to buy clothes, but she still enjoys window shopping and looking at the latest fashions.

Wing it

To perform to the best of one's ability in a circumstance for which one is not prepared.

When Wendy was out of town, Charmaine had to wing it at the board meeting.

Wipe the floor with (someone or something)

To defeat something or someone in a competition, or to physically harm someone.

The new arthritis drug wiped the floor clean with the COX-2 inhibitor.

Wipe the slate clean

To begin again without regard to previous events.

Based on his psychologist's advice, Charlie wanted to wipe the slate clean and establish a better relationship with his parents.

Wishful thinking

To hope for something that has little chance of happening.

Gina's oncologist told her that her cancer was so advanced that remission was little more than wishful thinking.

With a heavy heart

Sadly.

With a heavy heart, the surgeon told the patient's family that he hadn't survived the operation.

With bells on

Eagerly, enthusiastically.

When Dr. Nestor asked Jaime to come in next week for a followup visit, he said he'd be there with bells on.

With everything on it

To include every available condiment.

Marge ordered her hamburger with mustard and pickles only, but Carrie asked for her burger with everything on it.

With flying colors

Easily and exceptionally.

Khryss passed her state medical licensing exam with flying colors.

With it

Alert and conversant.

The EMTs reported that the patient wasn't with it when they arrived on the scene, and the emergency department doctors confirmed that he was still confused and incoherent at the time of his arrival at the hospital.

With no strings attached

To be free of hidden agendas or stipulations.

Marvin's counselor offered him three months of free sessions with no strings attached.

With one hand tied behind (one's) back

To perform an action with ease, even under exceptionally difficult conditions.

Dr. Johnson can set a broken bone with one hand tied behind his back.

With (one's) tail between (one's) legs

To be ashamed.

When David's teacher caught him in a lie, he ran out of the classroom with his tail between his legs.

With regard to (someone or something)

To speak in reference to something or someone.

Dr. Culpepper wanted to speak to the patient with regard to his treatment plan.

With relish

Enthusiastically.

Bonnie started her physical therapy with relish.

Within a stone's throw

To be very close to something.

We were within a stone's throw of the accident.

Within an inch of (one's) life

Close to death.

The patient was taken to the OR just in time: He was within an inch of his life.

Within reason

To cautiously acknowledge potential limitations.

The nurse told the patient he could resume his normal activities, within reason.

Within walking distance

A place that is close enough to travel to on foot.

The hematology lab was within walking distance of the outpatient clinic.

Without fail

Dependably and with no exceptions.

An updated lab report must be on the chart this afternoon without fail.

Without further ado

Promptly; with no additional interruption.

After getting a brief update on the accident victim's vital statistics, the emergency room doctor began treating her without further ado.

Without question

With certainty.

Without question, if the patient does not go through rehab, he will not regain use of his leg.

Without rhyme or reason

To lack coherence.

There was no rhyme or reason to the departmental procedures.

Woe is me

Said when one is feeling sorry for oneself.

Brittany expressed such self-pity during her session that her counselor was surprised that she didn't come in saying, "Woe is me."

Word to the wise

Good advice.

Here is a word to the wise: Follow your doctor's orders and stay fit.

Words to that effect

To paraphrase a statement.

The doctor said that Liza's condition was terminal, or words to that effect.

Work wonders

To produce dramatic beneficial effects.

Taking a walk each day works wonders for the circulatory system.

Worked up

Excited or agitated about something.

The patient got worked up over the change in the treatment plan.

Worth its weight in gold

Very valuable.

The Physician's Desk Reference is worth its weight in gold.

Wouldn't touch (something) with a ten-foot pole

To refuse to be involved with something under any circumstances.

Abby prefers to treat her emotional problems with psychotherapy and told her therapist that she wouldn't touch antidepressants with a 10-foot pole.

Wreak havoc

To cause a great deal of trouble.

The drug overdose wreaked havoc on the patient's nervous system.

Wrong side of the tracks

An undesirable, nonaffluent area.

Most people choose to go to the university hospital since the free clinic is on the wrong side of the tracks.

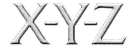

X-Y-Z

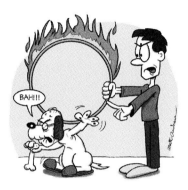

*You can't teach an
old dog new tricks*

X marks the spot

The exact place.

*Sally pointed to the location of her pain and told the
doctor that X marks the spot.*

Year in and year out

Continually; every year.

I get hay fever year in and year out.

Yield the right-of-way

To defer to someone or something else.

The ER team deals with many accidents caused by someone failing to yield the right-of-way at a crosswalk or stop sign.

You bet your boots

Surely, absolutely.

You bet your boots the pharmaceutical company wants the FDA to approve its new Alzheimer drug.

You can bet on it

You can be sure that this will take place.

The doctor will prescribe amoxicillin for Bobby's ear infection – you can bet on it.

You can't take it with you

Enjoy one's resources while one is living, because material wealth does not transcend death.

Jean didn't have any concerns about paying the high price for a facelift: She knows you can't take it with you.

You can't teach an old dog new tricks

Inability to impart wisdom to someone because of his or her preestablished routine or mindset.

The nurse tried to show Hal how to use the new digital glucose monitor, but he told her he preferred his usual method, saying, "You can't teach an old dog new tricks."

Your guess is as good as mine

To have no knowledge of something.

I am not sure when the patient will be discharged:
Your guess is as good as mine.

Your secret is safe with me

To promise to keep a confidence.

I know you've ignored the doctor's orders not to eat
fried food, but your secret is safe with me.

Zero in on (something)

To focus on something.

Dr. Riley zeroed in on Jimmy's abdominal pain.

Zonk out

To fall into a deep sleep.

Patients usually zonk out after only a few minutes
under anesthesia.

Zoom in on (something)

To focus on something.

Dr. Harris wanted to zoom in on the patient's chief
complaint of chest pain.